Substance Use and Misuse in sub-Saharan Africa

Magen Mhaka-Mutepfa
Editor

Substance Use and Misuse in sub-Saharan Africa

Trends, Intervention, and Policy

palgrave
macmillan

Editor
Magen Mhaka-Mutepfa
Department of Psychology, Faculty of Social Sciences
University of Botswana
Gaborone, Botswana

ISBN 978-3-030-85731-8 ISBN 978-3-030-85732-5 (eBook)
https://doi.org/10.1007/978-3-030-85732-5

This Palgrave Macmillan imprint is published by the registered company Springer Nature Switzerland AG.
The registered company address is: Gewerbestrasse 11, 6330 Cham, Switzerland

This book is dedicated to all members of our extended families, friends, colleagues, and young people currently grappling with substance use disorders.

Acknowledgements

The aim of the project was to get a multidisciplinary team working in the field of substance use/misuse who understand how it is defined, experienced, and treated to share their knowledge. The team was made up of authors from the health sciences, psychiatry, social sciences, hospitals, private practices, and non-governmental organizations that deal with substance use/misuse issues. The editor is indebted to Associate Professor Bontle Mbongwe and Dr. James January for assisting with conceptualization and reviewing of the book. The Editor extends her gratitude to Professor Seth Oppong who reviewed the whole book. Sincere gratitude also goes to Ms Leonne Mfolwe who reviewed and formatted all the book chapters. The editor also wishes to acknowledge a few colleagues who were not part of the project but helped review some of the book chapters. They include Lorato Kenosi, Mondy Segopolo, and Boitumelo Vavani. I acknowledge Mpho Pheko, K. Manyanda and all the other authors who helped review chapters in this book.

The authors benefited from the first National Tobacco Control Conference in 2017 organized by the Anti-Tobacco Network (Botswana) at Phakalane Hotel. International speakers and advocates at the conference spoke of the carnage of substance use, particularly tobacco, which was highlighted as a gateway substance to illicit drug use. The editor mulled the idea of teaching substance use and writing a prescribed book, of which some of the ideas originated from the conference presentations. Without the conference, this idea might not have been initiated and/or realized.

Contents

Notes on Contributors

James Ayugi is a senior mental health professional with vast experience in clinical psychiatry across the African continent spanning over three decades. Ayugi has previously worked with international organizations (UNDP) in Lesotho as a mental health advisor to the Government of Lesotho, and (United Nations) in Sierra Leone as team leader of the psychological team to the UN Mission in Freetown. Ayugi also served as colonel in the Kenya Defence Forces as Chief of Psychiatry before being appointed as the founding Head of Department of Psychiatry at Kenyatta University, Kenya. Dr Ayugi has authored books on *Mental Health and HIV in Lesotho* and *Horizons of Rape in Kenya*. Ayugi's academic interests include military psychiatry and substance use in military populations, medical education, rare psychiatric syndromes, and psychological trauma.

Wazha Dambe is a substance use disorder counsellor working at BOSASNet since 2011. He is an International Certified Addiction Professional (ICAP II). He is a member of the International Society of Substance Use Prevention and Treatment Professionals (ISSUP).

Kabo Diraditsile has an MSW and BSW from the University of Botswana. He is a PhD student at Waseda University in Japan. His interests are in social policy, substance use, and child and youth development issues. He has taught at the University of Botswana in the Department of Social Work, and has published extensively (chapters to books and refereed journal articles) on substance use/misuse and mental health among the youth in Botswana. He has presented papers at numerous international conferences and workshops; he also sits on editorial boards of two international journals.

Ketwesepe Hendrick is an interning psychological counsellor at the University of Botswana Psychology department. She has a Bachelor's degree in Psychology. Her research interests include substance use on young people and mental health awareness. Her graduate thesis was on the association between marijuana use and aggressive behaviour. Because of her passion for mental health, she engages with different populations to promote mental health and advocates for seeking psychological assistance.

James January is a public mental health practitioner and a senior lecturer and chair of the Department of Community Medicine at the University of Zimbabwe. Dr January has over 20 years of experience in mental health practice and research. His background is in psychology, with specific training and expertise in mental health and public health. Dr January has vast experience in survey research methods and secondary data analysis related to public health issues. He has written extensively On these topics and his research interests include mental health promotion in resource-limited settings and how psychological disorders such as substance use disorders impact on communities.

Refilwe Precious Jeremiah Bachelor of Social Work (BSW), Master in Social Work (MSW) is a senior lecturer in the Department of Social Work at the University of Botswana. She has earned a Master's degree in Social Work (specializing in mental health) with an emphasis on substance use/misuse from the University of Utah, USA. She has extensively published research and presented in international conferences on alcohol misuse issues. Some of her published work includes Alcohol Misuse and Intervention Strategies in Botswana: A Preliminary Study, and Alcohol and Poverty in Botswana.

Thabo Katlholo is the programs manager for the Anti Tobacco Network—a civil society organization based at the University of Botswana specializing in tobacco control advocacy, training on tobacco control, research, education, and awareness on tobacco-related issues. He holds a Bachelor's Degree in Biological Sciences from the University of Botswana. He has certification in Project Management from the University of Stellenbosch Business School and holds an MSc in Project Management from the University of Bolton, UK.

Ability C. Katsidzira is currently a registered pharmacist working at Edendale Hospital. She has eight years of experience in dispensing medications to people in KwaZulu-Natal with various medical conditions. She often interacts with patients misusing prescription drugs. Her current research interest is on use/misuse of medicine from medical prescriptions. Working at one of the biggest tertiary institutions in a rural setting in KwaZulu-Natal-South Africa with a big catchment area has exposed her to a plethora of cases of patients misusing medications due to different reasons.

Tshephiso Theodora Khame is an intern at the University of Botswana Psychology Clinic. She obtained her Bachelor's degree, majoring in Psychology and Sociology in 2019 and has also been a teaching assistant at the department. She is gaining clinical experience through supervision by registered clinical psychologists. She has helped professors facilitate mental health workshops and discussions in secondary schools and tertiary institutions.

Rachel W. Kimani is a lecturer of nursing at the Aga Khan University, Kenya. She joined the School of Nursing and Midwifery (SONAM), Kenya, in 2019 and currently teaches pathophysiology, research, and advanced nursing concepts. Dr Kimani also chairs the SONAM Kenya research committee, coordinates research in the department, and represents the department in various campus committees. She has previously worked at the Rockefeller University in New York as a clinical researcher in the Laboratory of the Biology of Addictive Diseases. As a scholar, her interests are mental health, women's health, building research capacity in primary health care, advanced nursing practice, and policy implications for universal health coverage.

Katlego Lone Maikano is a psychological counsellor and psychometric assistant at the Legato Center for Psychometric Assessment in Botswana. She graduated from the University of Botswana in 2020, with a Bachelor's Degree in Psychology. She is pursuing her Master's degree in Psychology and her research interest is in substance use.

David Sidney Mangwegape is a lecturer in Psychiatric Mental Health Nursing, a GCCE credentialed Addiction Professional (International Certified Addiction Professional [ICAP II]) and a psychiatric mental health nurse with over 17 years experience. He is passionate about mental health and dependence issues leading him to play an advocacy role that culminated in the establishment of a mental health awareness NGO called Embrace Emotions Support Network (EESN) that he co-founded in 2016. He anchors a column "The Mental Health Series" in the Midweek Sun newspaper in Botswana since February 2018. He is also the author of a self-published mental health promotion book "Gateways to Better Mental Health."

Kegomoditswe Manyanda is a clinician, lecturer, and researcher, currently working in private practice (Aspire Health Services Group). Manyanda is a registered clinical psychologist and holds a Master's Degree in Clinical Psychology from Roosevelt University in Chicago, USA. She is a certified addiction professional holding an International Certified Addiction Professional II (ICAP II). She has over 16 years of experience working in the field of mental health both in hospital and outpatient settings, including at the Botswana Substance Abuse Support Network (BOSASNet). She has spearheaded a number of substance abuse prevention campaigns and has worked with a number of stakeholders. She is also a member of the International Society of Substance Use Prevention and Treatment Professionals (ISSUP).

Kesego Mathoothe is a counselling psychologist registered with the Botswana Health Professions Council. She works as a part-time lecturer at the Institute of Development Management in Botswana. She teaches psychology courses including substance use at the tertiary institution.

Bontle Mbongwe is an associate professor in the Department of Environmental Sciences at the University of Botswana and a founder member of an NGO called anti-tobacco network, whose sole purpose is to fully implement government obligations in tobacco control. The NGO has attracted lots of funding for Botswana. She has won UN and WHO awards for her work on tobacco control. Whilst working at the Ministry of Health, she has contributed to several policy guidelines in the areas of chemical safety, tobacco control, and public health. Additionally she has attracted external funding for research on alcohol and tobacco use as principal investigator in several projects running concurrently.

Leonne Mfolwe is a teaching assistant at the University of Botswana where she facilitates psychology courses. She is an industrial psychologist registered with the Botswana Health Professions Council. Her major research interest is health and wellness, particularly with regard to mental health challenges, including substance use disorders.

Farai A. Mhaka is a registered pharmacist with the South African Pharmacy Council since 2013. He is currently working at Edendale Hospital and has six years of experience in dispensing medicines. Medicines dispensed range from acute treatment to chronic therapies for several conditions. Mhaka's work focuses on rational use of medicines, evaluation of prescription medicines, and, if need be, provides pharmacist-initiated therapy and hence, the interest on misuse of medicines from medical prescriptions.

Magen Mhaka-Mutepfa is an associate professor in the Department of Psychology, Faculty of Social Sciences at the University of Botswana. She teaches psychology and public health courses inclusive of substance use/misuse. Previously she was a teaching assistant in the School of Public Health at the University of Sydney (New South Wales (NSW)), and was a recipient of the Australia International Postgraduate Research Scholarship and Australian Postgraduate Award. Prior to attaining a doctoral degree, she worked as coordinator counsellor at the University of Zimbabwe. She was also employed as a guidance and counselling officer in the Ministry of Education, Sport and Culture in Zimbabwe where she championed advocacy on HIV/AIDs and substance use/misuse. She is a registered psychologist with more than ten years of cross-discipline experience in psychotherapy support services, more than ten years of teaching experience, and has also worked as a research consultant for the Pacific Institute of Research and Evaluation (four years).

Refilwe Pearl Mogomotsi is an intern and teaching assistant in the Department of Psychology at the University of Botswana. She has a Bachelor's degree in Social Sciences, majoring in Psychology and Sociology at the University of Botswana. She completed two research papers during her undergraduate studies on Knowledge of Improved HIV Treatment and the Likelihood of Engaging in Risky Sexual Behaviours among Students and on Perceptions of Student's Safety in the University of Botswana. She has since volunteered at Stepping Stones International as a mentor and also volunteers at Teen Spirit as a teen mentor.

Keneilwe Molebatsi is a psychiatrist and senior lecturer at the University of Botswana. She graduated with a Bachelor of Medicine and Surgery degree from the University of KwaZulu Natal (UKZN) in South Africa and holds a Master of Medicine in Psychiatry from the University of Nairobi in Kenya. She is currently pursuing a PhD in Psychiatry at UKZN focusing on trauma in patients with severe mental illness. Dr Molebatsi's other research interests include child and adolescent mental health, with a special interest in the association between exposure to childhood adversity and negative psychological outcomes such as substance use and interventions to improve recognition and management of depression across all levels of health care.

Anthony Olashore has a broad background in psychiatry, with training and expertise in adolescent mental health and drug use. His current research interest includes mental health in adolescents living with HIV. He has conducted research and published articles on drug use/misuse among university students. He has an ongoing project on substance use and mental disorders in secondary school students. His PhD topic is on the association of substance use, mental illness, cognition, and Highly Active Antiretroviral Therapy (HAART) adherence in HIV-infected adolescents in Botswana.

Philip Opondo is currently assistant programme director in the Department of Psychiatry at the University of Botswana and an adjunct assistant professor of psychiatry at the Perelman School of Medicine, Pennsylvania, USA. He has worked in the mental health field for over 25 years. His research interests are in stigma, HIV/AIDS and mental health, transcultural psychiatry, and substance use/misuse. He has published two books on psychiatry and has over 20 publications to his credit, including topics related to substance use.

Seth Oppong PhD, Member of Ghana Psychological Association (MGPA) is an associate professor at the Department of Psychology, University of Botswana. He obtained his doctorate from the University of Ghana, Legon. He is a member of the Ghana Psychological Association and Global Organisation for Humanitarian Work Psychology. He was an international visiting research scholar at North Carolina State University, Raleigh, and a Carnegie Scholar at the University of Ghana, Legon. His research interests include meta-science with respect to psychology; public (sector) psychology; psychotechnics; and indigenous occupational health. He has published in the areas of occupational health and taught occupational health and safety as well as human factors in the work environment. He has also been involved in corporate consulting on workplace psychosocial hazard assessment and interventions in the financial and brewing industries.

Mpho M. Pheko is an associate professor and Head of the Psychology Department at the University of Botswana. She has experience heading an academic department in a university setting, as well as consulting experience designing and implementing business strategies, training and development programmes, and change management programmes. She also has experience supervising research, leading research teams, and publishing academic work. Her research interests include "labor market issues," "public psychology," "dysfunctional organizational behaviours and practices," and "youth development" amongst others. She has written papers in the areas of youth development, workplace bullying and mobbing, and employment creation.

Shathani Rampa has supervised student research projects on the different effects of marijuana use on university students in Botswana. She is also a member of the Committee on Tobacco Dependence and Cessation as well as the Committee on Research, Monitoring and Evaluation in the Anti-Tobacco Network in Botswana. She was also a member of the organizing committee at the third Africa and Middle East Congress on Dependency (AMECA) hosted in Botswana in 2015.

Roy Tapera is a senior faculty member in the School of Public Health at the University of Botswana with ten years of experience. He is a public health specialist with extensive knowledge of epidemiology, health informatics, and health promotion. He has co-authored several papers on substance use and other public health issues. Dr Tapera is a board member of the Anti-Tobacco network, a non-governmental organization with a vision to have a tobacco-free Botswana. He is also an active member of the International Consortium of Universities for Drug Demand Reduction (ICUDDR).

Tshephiso Teseletso is a clinical psychologist. She does community work in the form of advocacy and community development and works with people of diverse backgrounds in healing trauma, depression, anxiety, addiction, as well as bringing together families. She is also a radio and TV host currently airing The Tales from Home show on YTV. Teseletso is an author and researcher in the field of psychiatry and mental health.

List of Figures

List of Tables

PART I

Risk Factors, Impact on Health, and Challenges

CHAPTER 1

Introductory Chapter

Magen Mhaka-Mutepfa

Abstract Substance use and misuse present a major public health risk and continues to affect younger populations in previously low use areas such as sub-Saharan Africa. With increased globalization, there has been an unprecedented increase in drug trafficking and acceptance of substance use/misuse, resulting in adverse consequences at the individual, family, community, and national levels. In this book, scholars from diverse behavioural sciences and public health disciplines analyze different issues surrounding substance use/misuse with an emphasis on sub-Saharan Africa. The introductory chapter covers concepts and use of terminology in substance use research and practice, including a section on epidemiology, while providing an overview of the whole book. The book is divided into two main sections with the first section (Chaps. 1, 2, 3, 4, 5, 6 and 7) emphasizing aetiology, signs and symptoms, risk factors, impact, and psychosocial challenges relating to use of conventional drugs, among others. The second section (Chaps. 8, 9, 10 and 11) focuses on prevention and intervention strategies to curtail substance use/misuse. Chap. 12 summarizes the book and suggests implications for research, practice, and policy.

M. Mhaka-Mutepfa (✉)
Department of Psychology, Faculty of Social Sciences, University of Botswana, Gaborone, Botswana
e-mail: mutepfam@ub.ac.bw

M. Mhaka-Mutepfa (ed.), *Substance Use and Misuse in sub-Saharan Africa*, https://doi.org/10.1007/978-3-030-85732-5_1

The book is inspired by the evidently increasing substance use as a result of several factors which include, but are not limited to, stressful life events.

Keywords Substance use • Substance misuse • Sub-Saharan Africa • Terminology • Substance use disorders • Dependence

Substance use/misuse continues to have a great impact on public health in diverse settings and is a common phenomenon worldwide. The use and misuse of substances is also a major risk to mental illness (United Nations Office on Drugs and Crime (UNODC), 2018) and affects people, particularly younger populations, in previously low use areas such as sub-Saharan Africa (Diraditsile & Rasesigo, 2018). With increased globalization, there has been an unprecedented increase in drug trafficking and acceptance of substance use resulting in adverse consequences at the individual, family, community, and national levels. The situation is rife in Africa (Luengo-Cabrera & Moser, 2016) but the impact is not well known due to inadequate research, lack of advocacy, reporting, and intervention. Sky News (2021) reported that in England and Wales, the number of deaths related to alcohol use increased by almost 20% in 2020. Sky News also documented that about 80% of deaths related to alcohol use were from alcoholic liver disease, 10% from mental and behavioural disorders originating from alcohol use, and six (6%) from accidental poisoning by exposure to alcohol (Sky News, May 2021). The statistics are quite disconcerting given the fact that people have been grappling with containing COVID-19. Similar statistics are found in other countries throughout the world hence the need for advocacy, prevention, and effective intervention.

There is dearth of information on substance use in sub-Saharan Africa as researchers have been focusing mostly on communicable diseases, particularly HIV and AIDs and now COVID-19. Few published data/reports include surveys done on the prevalence of substance use in South Africa in 2012 (Peltzer & Phaswana-Mafuya, 2018) and 2018 (Kuteesa et al., 2019). Mortality rates resulting from substance use/misuse were also assessed in South Africa (Mouton et al., 2015). Nonetheless, there is also outdated information on concepts and approaches to sustainable community health with regard to substance use available to educators, policymakers, development agencies, and social service providers, even though community development and well-being are tied to community health (e.g., Institute of Medicine and National Academy of Sciences (IMNAS), 2010). Although the mortality rate due to substance use is reported to be higher in low- and middle-income countries (LMICs), research and statistics are limited when compared to high-income countries (Mouton et al., 2015; Peacock et al., 2018). Rigorous procedures for collection, collation, and reporting of data for precise assessments of substance use/misuse trends and its disease burden are a prerequisite (Peacock et al., 2018).

Substance use and misuse also lead to substance use disorders (SUDs) whereby affected individuals may lose control of their need to use a substance and become over-reliant. Further, substance use/misuse has deleterious effects on physical health (e.g., cancer, heart diseases, stroke, etc.), mental health (e.g., depression, anxiety, etc.), and may increase the likelihood of accidents and/or injury—hence the need for timely interventions. The current COVID-19 pandemic has exacerbated substance use/misuse problems as people are struggling with its negative physical, psychosocial, and economic effects, thereby calling for the bio-psychosocial model with regard to intervention and prevention. Studies in sub-Saharan Africa have revealed the need for advocacy and other public health interventions to curb this cumulative problem (e.g., Dada et al., 2018 in Nigeria; Kalema & Vanderplasschen, 2015 in South Africa; Idowu et al., 2018 in Uganda; Tapera et al., 2020 in Botswana), which is only possible if the impact of substance use is known.

Assessing the harmful effects of substance use poses numerous challenges. IMNAS (2010) recognized flaws emanating from using the disability-adjusted life years (DALYs) metric. For instance, its failure to include the psycho-social and/or economic influences at individual, family, societal, or health systems levels or the real burden that substance use and misuse has on the lives of victims and caregivers. Acknowledging the aforementioned limitations on a DALYs and years-living-with-disability (YLDs) basis, this book will make use of the bio-psychosocial model to understand the impact of substance use, misuse, treatment, and intervention strategies in sub-Saharan Africa even though Africa has the lowest disease burden (DALYs=4%; YLDs=18%) due to having less neuropsychiatric ailments than the rest of the world (DALYs=12%; YLDs=31%) (IMNAS, 2010). Neuropsychiatric ailments (e.g., dependences, depression) result from traumatic brain injury which is mostly caused by alcohol and other substance use, and environmental influences. Nonetheless, psychological and psychiatric treatments reduce the inception of use, enhancing the significance of this book.

In the current book, scholars from different countries explore contemporary issues concerning the use and misuse of substances. The book focuses on the physical, cultural, and psychological/emotional aspects of substance use (e.g., dependence), its impact on health and the populace, prevention, treatment, and intervention.

Aims and Scope of the Book

The topics covered in this book are of immense interest to students, academics, health personnel, and researchers in medical, social, and behavioural sciences. This book will give an exposition of use and misuse of substances and it can be used by students of psychology, social work, public health, pharmacy, and psychiatry. The focus is on advocacy, the best approaches to intervene and curtail substance use and misuse. The book may also be of interest to policymakers, civil society, and other stakeholders interested in raising awareness or developing interventions on substance use and misuse. It further seeks to provide a resource on sustainable community health concepts, procedures, and practices for addressing substance use for the health and well-being of partner communities. Alcohol, tobacco, marijuana, and prescription drugs are the most commonly misused substances across age groups; however, the use pattern of the aforementioned and other drugs and their impact vary depending on life stage (Schulte & Hser, 2014). The foregoing authors posited that in terms of health outcomes, all ages are at risk for overdose, accidental injury, and intended injury such as suicide.

Concerning prevention and intervention: behavioural, environmental, psychosocial, and cultural factors that may affect substance use are addressed and applied to various aspects of use; for instance, dependence, intoxication, and withdrawal on substances such as tobacco, alcohol, marijuana, and others. This book could not have come at any other opportune time. The advent of COVID-19 has led to an increase in substance use (Wang et al., 2021). In addition to other risks arising from substance use, those with SUDs are more likely to develop COVID-19 and experience worse COVID-19 outcomes, including a higher risk of hospitalization and mortality (Wang et al., 2021). The aforementioned authors also posited that the impact is further affected by disparities in access to healthcare in different communities.

Rassool (2018) and Winger et al. (2004) are important sources of literature on substance use. However, they provide a more general approach to substance use and in many cases speak to a Western rather than African audience. Winger et al. (2004), for instance, took a more biomedical approach, while Rassool (2018) took a multidisciplinary approach. The current book project distinguishes itself from these books in terms of providing evidence and practices from a diverse perspective, particularly the perspectives from the non-Western, Educated, Industrialized, Rich, and Democratic (non-WEIRD) contexts. Though this book also takes a multidisciplinary approach, it differs from Rassool's book because the book benefits from the expertise of different specialists; Rassool's book was authored by a single expert placing limitations on the extent of knowledge that can be shared in each chapter. Similarly, this book differs from Winger et al.'s book given that the former was written with a non-technical audience in mind. This book project seeks to create literature that will support the training of and practice by health and dependence practitioners in international contexts. The book project will also provide a much-needed context-specific and context-relevant literature for teachers, students, and practitioners in non-Western contexts.

The book by Ndasauka and Kayange (2019) is an exception, although its focus was on dependence. It is a vital source of literature and prevalence of dependency in African settings. The prevalence of dependence is a good starting point as it helps students and practitioners design effective psychoeducation programs for clients. However, while it might have incorporated the bio-psychosocial model, the book focused on dependence and offered a more general approach to substance use.

Contributors of the current book have also focused on challenges experienced by users and how to prevent, promote, and intervene with regard to substance use/misuse. Change is complex and context-specific and differs across cultures; therefore, readers should take cognizance of the types of interventions implemented. Several questions have guided the editor and the chapter authors. These include:

1. What are the burdens of diseases in sub-Saharan Africa?
2. How do SUDs manifest as developmental disorders?
3. What are the causes, risk factors, signs, and symptoms of mental and behavioural disorders?
4. What is the impact of substance use/misuse on non-communicable and communicable diseases such as HIV/AIDS and COVID-19?

5. What is the impact of tobacco advertising and promotion on youth smoking in developing countries?
6. What strategies are used to reduce tobacco advertising and promotion using the Framework Convention on Tobacco Control (FCTC) as a proven tool?
7. What significant socio-economic losses are attributed to the harmful use of substances, particularly alcohol?
8. What are the theoretical models underpinning the revolution of substance use?
9. How do the alcohol industry and its policies impact substance use?
10. What is the impact of harmful substances on health?
11. How does the introduction of prescription drugs to Africa increase the availability and misuse of psychoactive substances?
12. How does substance use affect work performance and organizational productivity?
13. What measures can be used to reduce substance use, particularly among the youth?
14. Which prevention and intervention strategies are effective in curtailing substance use in adults?

Sections of the Book

This book was inspired by the number of young people who experience adverse drug reactions and died from substance use and misuse including prescription drugs (see Klein et al., 2020; Mbongwe et al., 2020; Mouton et al., 2015). Morbidity and mortality have motivated us to take stock of challenges facing people in various contexts and countries. The world has many stressors; poverty, pandemics, abuse and stigma, bullying, and many others that need curtailing. In this book, scholars from different countries and diverse behavioural sciences and public health disciplines analyse different issues surrounding substance use/misuse with an emphasis on sub-Saharan Africa. Like other social groups, substance users are dynamic and subject to influences across their proximal and distal environments. Although people are subject to change over time, they retain characteristics from their past in their present hence the need for intervention. Users can be resilient and are capable of dealing with profound changes if provided with the requisite support.

The introductory chapter covers concepts and use of terminology in substance use research and practices while providing an overview of the whole book. The book is divided into two main sections with the first section (Chaps. 1, 2, 3, 4, 5, 6 and 7) emphasizing aetiology, signs and symptoms, risk factors, impact, and psychosocial challenges relating to the use of conventional drugs, among others. The second section (Chaps. 8, 9, 10, 11 and 12) focuses on substance use in the workplace, misuse of prescription drugs, treatment, prevention, and intervention strategies to curb substance use. Each chapter comprises case studies and follow-up questions for practice and reflection. Case studies identifying problems with substance use are presented to provide a more robust discussion. The two sections integrate and synthesize many of the most important issues affecting substance use, misuse, prevention, treatment, and intervention.

Chapter 2 explores early developmental influences on substance use disorders; it embraces a developmental perspective in reviewing the underlying mechanisms of SUDs. This developmental perspective provides a holistic view of SUDs as a process, highlighting the interaction of multiple contributory factors over the lifespan. Prominent models of SUDs are also discussed.

Chapter 3 examines alcohol use. A focus on alcohol use/misuse is important as the World Health Organization (WHO, 2018) attributes 5.1% of the global burden of disease and injury to the use of alcohol. Alcohol is the most extensively used and misused substance throughout the world. Beyond health consequences, the harmful use of alcohol is attributed to major socio-economic losses to individuals, families, and societies. Aetiology, risk factors, signs, and symptoms of mental and behavioural disorders attributed to alcohol are explored. Chapter 4 presents a summary of the policies and laws that control and mitigate the use of alcohol, using examples from different countries in sub-Saharan Africa. The antagonistic marketing and policy meddling actions by alcohol producers, some of which are criticized by civil society and public health campaigners are also discussed.

Chapter 5 analyzes tobacco as a looming epidemic in sub-Saharan Africa. The chapter highlights the epidemiology of tobacco use and exposure to tobacco smoke, which are said to exacerbate the prevalence of non-communicable and communicable diseases. The detrimental impact of tobacco use on people's health is also explored, suggesting that tobacco use should be a public health priority. Chapter 6 gives an exposition of the

WHO Framework Convention on Tobacco Control (FCTC). The WHO FCTC is the first global evidence-based public health treaty developed by countries in response to the pandemic use of tobacco products and the aggressive tactics of the tobacco industry that undermine public health efforts (WHO, 2005). This chapter explores the catalytic role the FCTC has played globally in curbing tobacco use since its adoption in 2003. Measures relating to the reduction of demand and supply of tobacco in sub-Saharan Africa are discussed. Chapter 7 explores the most commonly used illicit drugs (e.g., cocaine, heroin, marijuana, whoonga, etc.) and their effect on health and wellbeing. Factors that lead to the use of illicit drugs are discussed. The effect each substance has on the physical and mental health of individuals and communities is also debated, including resultant diseases.

Chapter 8 of the second section emphasizes substance use in organizations, policies, and interventions. Counterproductive work behaviours related to substance use such as lateness, absenteeism, presenteeism (physically present but unproductive), workplace incivilities, psychosomatic ailments, as well as physical ailments are discussed. Policymakers, human resources practitioners, unions, and other stakeholders are encouraged to take cognizance of the harmful impact of substance use during working hours or otherwise and make appropriate interventions.

Chapter 9 elucidates prescription drug misuse and prevention strategies. There is anecdotal evidence that prescription drug misuse is a major global concern particularly in low and middle-income countries (LMICs). This problem only comes to light when well-known personalities (celebrities) die from prescription drug misuse. The three most commonly misused psychoactive prescription drugs, that is, stimulants (e.g. methamphetamine), opioids (e.g. codeine), and central nervous system depressants (e.g. benzodiazepines) are discussed. Evidence-based prevention strategies, harm reduction, and current treatment interventions for prescription drug disorders are also explored in this chapter.

Chapter 10 examines the prevention of SUDs in special populations (e.g., poor or homeless, young adults or teenagers, the elderly and trauma survivors). Special populations have unique health concerns that require extraordinary attention in the prevention and treatment of SUDs. Young people's engagement with substances, challenges, best practices, and recommendations for prevention and treatment are also presented. Chapter

11 takes cognizance of the fact that there is no single approach to dealing with substance use as intervention depends on aetiology, personality traits of the users, and the different rehabilitation institutions, while exploring the effective prevention and intervention strategies of substance use in adults. The following interventions are discussed: cognitive-based therapies, confrontational models of intervention, crisis intervention, systemic family models of persuasive intervention, and school-based prevention education intervention. Chapter 12 concludes the book and is inspired by the increasing substance use/misuse because of several factors which include but are not limited to stressful life events.

Readers should take cognizance that when distressed individuals are able to recover, they operate from a foundation of strength and can, therefore, perform their roles with greater efficacy. The use of illicit and licit substances is a cause for concern and may lead to harm hence the need for prevention. The provision of more qualified specialists to intervene is needed in sub-Saharan countries to combat the rising numbers of substance use cases in both adolescents and adults. Nonetheless, certain terms are discouraged from use to evade and reduce stigma when writing about substance use/misuse.

Stigmatizing Words to Avoid, Words to Use, and Definitions

While certain language may be considered disparaging, it is generally used within social communities of people who struggle with SUDs. Feeling stigmatized can reduce the willingness of individuals with SUDs to seek treatment (Yang et al., 2017), and stigmatizing language can negatively influence healthcare providers' perceptions of people with SUDs (Ashford et al., 2019), which can impact the care they provide. Stigma can also reduce the readiness of policymakers to apportion resources, reduce the willingness of providers in non-specialty settings to screen for, and address substance use (Hadland et al., 2018). However, clinicians can demonstrate leadership in using acceptable language that may destigmatize words considered by stakeholders as inappropriate. The words and the definitions that may be used to destigmatize recurring concepts used in this book are given in Table 1.1. The words that are not defined in the table below will be explained in the respective chapters.

Table 1.1 Terms to avoid, terms to use and definitions

Terms to avoid	*Terms to use*	*Definitions*
Substance abuse (SA)	Substance use (for illicit drugs and licit drugs like alcohol and tobacco)	Is the harmful indulgence in substances for mood-altering purposes in a way that may pose a threat to health, families and even the community (Marshall & Spencer, 2018)
Substance abuse	Substance misuse (for prescription drugs)	Refers to occurrences or patterns of substance use not consistent with legal or medical guidelines and associated with physical, psychological, economic, and social problems (Schulte& Hser, 2014) It is also about the use of substances that may pose a risk to health, security or the well-being of individuals, families, or communities (Lander et al., 2013)
	Substance dependence and substance abuse are combined into SUDs in DSM (Diagnostic and Statistical Manual of Mental Disorders)-5 (American Psychiatric Association (APA), 2013)	SUDs are indicated by a problematic pattern of using any substance that results in impairment in daily life or other noticeable distress (Hartney & Gans, 2020)
Addiction	Dependence	'Negative consequences, (i.e., cravings, urges and the repetitive and excessive continued use of the substance) even when it disrupts a person's life, brought about by bio- psycho-social cultural factors' (Ndasauka & Kayange, 2019, p. 1)
	Substance dependence	This is indicated by a maladaptive pattern of substance use and misuse resulting in significant impairment or distress (Morrison, 2014)
	Tobacco use	Is defined as the use of any type of tobacco products, both smoked (consumption of smoke from burnt products) and smokeless (consumption of unburnt tobacco products by mouth or nose) (WHO, 2019)
Addict	Person with substance use disorder	
Alcoholic, drunk	Person with alcohol use disorder	Person who misuses alcohol

(*continued*)

Table 1.1 (continued)

Terms to avoid	*Terms to use*	*Definitions*
Substance or drug abuser, junkie	Patient	
Dirty	Testing positive for toxicology screen results	
Clean	Testing negative for toxicology screen results	

Adapted from the National Institute of Drug Abuse (May 2021).

References

American Psychiatric Association. (2013). *Diagnostic and statistical manual of mental disorders* (5th ed.). American Psychiatric Association.

Ashford, R. D., Brown, A. M., McDaniel, J., & Curtis, B. (2019). Biased labels: An experimental study of language and stigma among individuals in recovery and health professionals. *Substance Use & Misuse, 54*(8), 1376–1384. https://doi.org/10.1080/10826084.2019.1581221

Dada, S., Harker Burnhams, N., Laubscher, R., Parry, C., & Myers, B. (2018). Alcohol and other drug use among women seeking substance abuse treatment in the Western Cape, South Africa. *South African Journal of Science, 114*(9/10). https://doi.org/10.17159/sajs.2018/4451

Diraditsile, K., & Rasesigo, K. (2018). Substance abuse and mental health effects among the youth in Botswana: Implications for social research. *Journal of Education, Society and Behavioural Science, 24*(2), 1–11.

Hadland, S. E., Park, T. W., & Bagley, S. M. (2018). Stigma associated with medication treatment for young adults with opioid use disorder: A case series. *Addiction Science & Clinical Practice, 13*(1), 15. https://doi.org/10.1186/s13722-018-0116-2

Hartney, E., & Gans, S. (2020, March 21). *A guide to DSM 5 criteria for substance use disorders.* https://www.verywellmind.com/dsm-5-criteria-for-substance-use-disorders-21926

Idowu, A., Aremu, A. O., Olumide, A., & Ogunlaja, A. O. (2018). Substance abuse among students in selected secondary schools of an urban community of Oyo-state, southwest Nigeria: Implication for policy action. *African Health Sciences, 18*(3), 776–785. https://doi.org/10.4314/ahs.v18i3.36

Institute of Medicine and National Academy of Sciences. (2010). *Mental, neurological, and substance use disorders in sub-Saharan Africa: Reducing the treatment gap, improving quality of care. Summary of a joint workshop by the Institute of Medicine and the Uganda National Academy of Sciences.* The National Academies Press. https://doi.org/10.17226/12828

Kalema, D., & Vanderplasschen, W. (2015). Features and challenges of alcohol abuse treatment in Uganda. *African Journal of Drug & Alcohol Studies, 14*(2), 125–135.

Klein, A., Patwardhan, S., & Loglo, M. G. A. (2020). Divergences and commonalities between the US opioid crisis and prescription medicine mis/use in West Africa. *International Journal of Drug Policy, 76*, 102640.

Kuteesa, M. O., Seeley, J., Weiss, H. A., Cook, S., Kamali, A., & Webb, E. L. (2019). Alcohol misuse and illicit drug use among occupational groups at high risk of HIV in sub-Saharan Africa: A systematic review. *AIDS and Behavior, 23*(12), 3199–3225.

Lander, L., Howsare, J., & Byrne, M. (2013). The impact of substance use disorders on families and children: From theory to practice. *Social Work in Public Health, 28*(3-4), 194–205. https://doi.org/10.1080/19371918.2013.759005

Luengo-Cabrera, J., & Moser, A. (2016). Transatlantic drug trafficking-via Africa. *European Union Institute for Security Studies, 3*, 1–2.

Marshall, B., & Spencer, J. (2018). *Essentials of substance use disorders.* Springer Publishing Company.

Mbongwe, B., Moinami, J., Masupe, T., Tapera, R., Molefe, T., Erick, P., Godman, B., & Massele, A. (2020). Nature and sources of poisoning in patients admitted to a referral hospital in Gaborone, Botswana; Findings and implications. *Hospital Practice, 48*(2), 100–107.

Morrison, J. (2014). *DSM-5 made easy- The clinician's guide to diagnosis.* The Guilford Press.

Mouton, J. P., Mehta, U., Parrish, A. G., Wilson, D. P., Stewart, A., Njuguna, C. W., Kramer, N., Maartens, G., Blockman, M., & Cohen, K. (2015). Mortality from adverse drug reactions in adult medical inpatients at four hospitals in South Africa: A cross-sectional survey. *British Journal of Clinical Pharmacology, 80*(4), 818–826.

National Institute of Drug Abuse. (2021, May 25). *Words matter – Terms to use and avoid when talking about addiction.* https://www.drugabuse.gov/nidamed-medical-health-professionals/health-professions-education/words-matter-terms-to-use-avoid-when-talking-about-addiction

Ndasauka, Y., & Kayange, G. M. (Eds.). (2019). *Dependency in South and East Africa: Interdisciplinary approaches.* Palgrave Macmillan/Springer.

Peacock, A., Leung, J., Larney, S., Colledge, S., Hickman, M., Rehm, J., Giovino, G. A., West, R., Hall, W., Griffiths, P., Ali, R., Gowing, L., Marsden, J., Ferrari, A. J., Grebely, J., Farrell, M., &Degenhardt, L. (2018). Global statistics on alcohol, tobacco and illicit drug use: 2017 status report. *Addiction (Abingdon, England), 113*(10), 1905–1926. https://doi.org/10.1111/add.14234

Peltzer, K., & Phaswana-Mafuya, N. (2018). Drug use among youth and adults in a population-based survey in South Africa. *South African Journal of Psychiatry, 24.*

Rassool, H. (2018). *Alcohol and drug misuse: A guide for health and social care professionals* (2nd ed.). Routledge.

Schulte, M. T., & Hser, Y. I. (2014). Substance use and associated health conditions throughout the lifespan. *Public Health Reviews, 35*(2). https://doi.org/10.1007/BF03391702

Sky News. (2021, May 6). *Alcohol deaths highest for 20 years in England and Wales.* https://news.sky.com/story/alcohol-deaths-highest-for-20-years-in-england-and-wales-new-data-shows-12298375

Tapera, R., Mbongwe, B., Mhaka-Mutepfa, M., Lord, A., Phaladze, N. A., & Zetola, N. M. (2020). The theory of planned behavior as a behavior change model for tobacco control strategies among adolescents in Botswana. *PLoS ONE, 15*(6). https://doi.org/10.1371/journal.pone.0233462

United Nations Office on Drugs and Crime. (2018). *World drug report.* United Nations Office on Drugs and Crime. https://www.unodc.org/wdr2018/index.html

Wang, Q. Q., Kaelber, D. C., Xu, R., & Volkow, N. D. (2021). COVID-19 risk and outcomes in patients with substance use disorders: Analyses from electronic health records in the United States. *Molecular Psychiatry, 26*, 30–39. https://doi.org/10.1038/s41380-020-00880-7

Winger, G., Woods, J. H., & Hofmann, F. (2004). *A handbook on drug and alcohol misuse: The biomedical aspects* (4th ed.). Oxford University Press.

World Health Organisation. (2018). *Global status report on alcohol and health.* World Health Organisation. https://apps.who.int/iris/handle/10665/274603

World Health Organisation. (2019). *WHO report on the global tobacco epidemic, 2019: Offer help to quit tobacco use.* World Health Organisation. https://www.who.int/teams/health-promotion/tobacco-control/who-report-on-the-global-tobacco-epidemic-2019

World Health Organization. (2005). *WHO framework convention on tobacco control.* World Health Organization. https://www.who.int/tobacco/framework/WHO_FCTC_english.pdf

Yang, L. H., Wong, L. Y., Grivel, M. M., & Hasin, D. S. (2017). Stigma and substance use disorders: An international phenomenon. *Current Opinion in Psychiatry, 30*(5), 378–388. https://doi.org/10.1097/YCO.0000000000000351

CHAPTER 2

Aetiology and Early Developmental Influences on Substance Use Disorders

Shathani Rampa, Keneilwe Molebatsi, and James January

Abstract Adverse childhood experiences (ACEs) and psychosocial adversities in adolescence have been associated with an increase in substance use disorders (SUDs). Understanding ACEs, and environmental and psychological factors associated with these disorders is imperative in designing and implementing appropriate interventions to address SUDs. This chapter adopts a developmental perspective to review the underlying mechanisms of SUDs. Whereas early models of SUDs such as the brain disease model, social learning theory, and the moral model provide a useful base for understanding the mechanisms involved in the aetiology of these

S. Rampa • K. Molebatsi
University of Botswana, Gaborone, Botswana
e-mail: srampa@gradcenter.cuny.edu; molebatsik@ub.ac.bw

J. January (✉)
Department of Community Medicine, College of Health Sciences, University of Zimbabwe, Harare, Zimbabwe
e-mail: jamesj@medsch.uz.ac.zw

M. Mhaka-Mutepfa (ed.), *Substance Use and Misuse in sub-Saharan Africa*, https://doi.org/10.1007/978-3-030-85732-5_2

conditions, recent models of SUDs have adopted multimodal and developmental SUDs approaches which emphasise the role of experiences of adversity at key stages of development. The main advantage of the multimodal and developmental perspective is that it offers a holistic view of SUDs as a process, highlighting the interaction of multiple contributory factors over the lifespan. This chapter, therefore, explores prominent models of SUDs, and the role of different biological, social, and psychological factors during childhood and adolescence in the development and maintenance of SUDs.

Keywords Developmental influences • Brain disease model • Social learning theory • Dependence • Neurobiological factors • Psychosocial challenges • Genetics • Substance use disorders

Early Models that Explain SUDs

Substance use disorders (SUDs) refer to the persistent use of substances such as alcohol and/or other drugs in a way that causes the individual to suffer clinically significant impairments related to physical and/or psychological health, as well as social and/or occupational functioning (American Psychiatric Association, 2013). Understanding SUDs, including the causes and effects, is critical for shaping public health policy and the development of effective treatments and interventions. Central to the debates surrounding SUDs is the question of agency: are SUDs a disease or a choice? The most prominent models, which are the brain disease model, the moral model, and the social learning theory will be briefly discussed below.

The Brain Disease Model of SUDs

The brain disease model postulates that SUDs are brain diseases which are caused by dysfunctional brain systems that are involved in reward and pleasure seeking. The model has dominated the discourse on SUDs although it has attracted a lot of controversy (Volkow et al., 2016; Volkow & Li, 2005). Over the last few decades there has been increasing evidence of the neurobiological correlates of SUDs (Volkow et al., 2016; Volkow & Li, 2005) with numerous studies indicating links between genetic, epigenetic, other neurobiological factors and the risk of SUDs. The model has contributed immensely to advances in effective psychopharmacological treatments and reduced stigma on those with SUDs through shifting the blame from the individual to viewing SUDs as a disease of the brain (Heather, 2017). Given that susceptibility to SUDs is different as people have a different genetic make-up and are exposed to varying environments as they age, there is need to explore how the brain disease model can be applied to those at different levels of development.

The Moral Model of SUDs

This model posits that the cause of SUDs is related to an individual's inherent moral weakness and lack of will power (Frank & Nagel, 2017). Whereas the brain disease model highlights dysfunctional neurobiological processes as the primary drivers of SUDs, the moral model emphasises personal choice. Proponents of the moral model state that the brain disease model is not adequate because it makes substance use/misuse an involuntary compulsion, whereas in most cases there is a conscious decision involved (Pickard, 2020). Substance use/misuse and morality have been closely entangled for centuries, where substance-related behaviours were gradually viewed as violations of societal values (Frank & Nagel, 2017). This view of SUDs as a personal weakness resulted in stigma, blame, and shame, thereby becoming significant barriers to treatment. To some extent, the model acknowledges the powerful influence that parental and societal roles may play in shaping a child and an adolescent's moral character which may be a risk or protective factor against SUDs. Nonetheless, the model shifted the public health focus and discourse from other factors that increase risk of SUDs, such as poverty and childhood maltreatment.

The Social Learning Theory of SUDs

The social learning model posits that SUDs are a result of behaviours learned from the environment. The social learning theory is often applied to various stages of SUDs, focusing on the cognitive processes involved in deviant behaviour (DeMartino et al., 2015; Krohn et al., 1985; Love et al., 2020; Niaura, 2000; Wilson, 1987, 1988). The theory has found firm footing in explaining the maintenance of SUDs through cravings, reinforcement of substance use behaviours, and differential association, where people learn their behaviours through their interactions with others (DeMartino et al., 2015; Krohn et al., 1985; Love et al., 2020; Niaura, 2000; Wilson, 1987, 1988). Although it is a very useful model, the social learning theory appears to have greater explanatory power for the use of 'soft substances' such as alcohol and cigarettes, than for 'hard' substances like cocaine and heroin (Kruis et al., 2020).

Recent Models that Explain SUDs

Early models of SUDs are criticised for taking a myopic approach to a multimodal issue (Hall et al., 2017). Later models have attempted to address this weakness by taking on a more holistic approach to understanding SUDs. One of those approaches is to frame SUDs as a developmental disorder. This model takes a biopsychosocial approach to understanding substance use/misuse, thereby considering the complex interaction between biological factors, psychological factors, and social factors associated with SUDs. Furthermore, the developmental lens emphasises both risk and protective factors in understanding the initiation and maintenance of substance use, as well as developing a substance use disorder.

The developmental approach is not an outright rejection of other models, but rather an integrative model that brings together elements of some of the already existing models and places them within a developmental framework. The developmental view of SUDs posits that people are exposed to the risk and protective factors for SUDs at a young age. Furthermore, people are most vulnerable to these factors during the stages of childhood and adolescence as their physiological, emotional, cognitive, and social systems are still undergoing growth and change processes which are key to healthy development (Hall et al., 2017; McCrory & Mayes, 2015; Sherr et al., 2014).

The Biopsychosocial Perspectives of SUDs

The following section will attempt to unpack the role of genetic, epigenetic, neurobiological, social and psychological risk and protective factors of SUDs. It is imperative to note that no single factor may be enough to explain how the disorders develop and that there is a constant interplay of different factors. During childhood and adolescence, a lot of rapid changes occur in an individual's physical, mental, social, and moral development and these all impact the risk of developing a SUD (Smith et al., 2016). For instance, children born to parents with SUDs experience pre- and post-natal challenges to their development such as disrupted foetal development (Mattson et al., 2019), emotional dysregulation, as well as potential neglect and abuse (Cicchetti & Handley, 2019). The social and psychological experiences of adversity affect neural functioning through the mechanisms of neuroplasticity and epigenetics, thereby increasing the risk of developing a SUD.

Role of Neurobiological Factors and Genetics in the Development of SUDs

The neurobiological risk and protective factors of SUDs include dysfunction and dysregulation in some brain areas and systems, neurotransmitter over- and under-activity, and genetic processes. Childhood and adolescence have critical periods of neural development and direct exposure to substances can change neural structure and functioning during these stages (Chambers et al., 2003; Feltenstein & See, 2008). The most relevant areas undergoing change during adolescence are associated with important psychosocial drivers of SUDs such as impulsivity, motivation, the stress response, and attachment (Chambers et al., 2003; Feltenstein & See, 2008). The interaction of these associated factors underlies the increased vulnerability to SUDs that is illustrated by the disproportionate rates of adolescent substance use/misuse as compared to other age groups.

However, the exact directionality of these interactions is yet to be determined. Although numerous brain areas have been associated with SUDs, the most studied are the amygdala and the frontal lobe. The amygdala is involved in conditioned learning, more specifically the stimulus-reward associations, which has been identified as one of the key mechanisms in the transition from casual substance use to developing a SUD, as well as relapse (Feltenstein & See, 2008; See et al., 2003) and is also implicated in arousal and stress responsivity which are linked to the maintenance of SUDs through negative reinforcement (Koob, 2009, 2017). Frontal lobe connectivity is one of the last phases of neural development that humans undergo and it is usually completed by the mid-twenties. The immaturity of the frontal lobe is associated with impulsivity, increased risky decision-making, and poor judgement, which are often touted as hallmarks of adolescence. These neuro-behavioural characteristics of adolescence increase vulnerability to experimentation with substances, especially when combined with other psychosocial factors such as peer pressure, adverse childhood experiences (ACEs) and other stressful life events during adolescence (Chambers et al., 2003). This system is a dopaminergic pathway and ACEs (such as childhood maltreatment and neglect) affect dopaminergic functioning by increasing dopamine sensitivity, thereby leading to stronger neurochemical responses to more salient stimuli such as substances.

Twin and family studies have found that SUDs are approximately 50% heritable (Volkow & Muenke, 2012). However, the challenge in genetic research has been isolating specific genes due to the polygenetic nature of SUDs. In addition, the study of environmental effects on gene expression (epigenetics) has provided insight on the possible multimodal mechanisms that increase risk for SUDs. The two primary epigenetic processes that have been studied are histone acetylation and histone methylation. These processes involve the activation or repression of genes and have been associated with various psychosocial correlates of SUDs, such as childhood neglect, maltreatment, and stress (Ajonijebu et al., 2017; Hamilton & Nestler, 2019; Pierce et al., 2018). The changes in genetic expression provide a link between the psychosocial factors and neurobiological factors, but also highlight the complex interactions that result in the inter-individual variability which colours SUDs.

Role of Child Neglect and Maltreatment in the Development of SUDs

ACEs are stressful or potentially traumatic events that occur during early life. ACEs comprise multiple forms of abuse, neglect and other environmental factors that can undermine the child's sense of safety and stability such as parental incarceration or mental illness. Epidemiological studies conducted in several African countries such as Kenya, Nigeria, Burkina Faso, Ghana, Malawi, and Uganda (Kabiru et al., 2010; Kiburi et al., 2018; Oladeji et al., 2010) have shown associations between adverse ACEs and SUDs in adolescence and adulthood. ACEs have also been reported to have a negative influence on the management of patients with SUDs.

Neglect and abuse have a strong association with decreased levels of oxytocin in the plasma, urine or cerebrospinal fluid (CSF). The reduced levels have been associated with impaired psychosocial functioning and reward-seeking behaviours which may predict substance use (Stockdale et al., 2007). In addition, childhood adversity alters dopamine-related neuronal activity and synaptic functions, and dopamine dysfunction is implicated in the pathophysiology of psychiatric disorders including depression and SUDs.

Role of Parental and/or Caregiver Substance Use on SUDs Development

Foetal exposure to substances is associated with negative birth outcomes, including impaired brain development (Caritis & Panigrahy, 2019; Carlier et al., 2020; Whiteman et al., 2014). Additionally, children who had perinatal exposure to substances are more likely to experience other adverse psychological and social factors thereby further increasing their risk of developing SUDs (Schempf, 2007). The effects of being raised by parents or caregivers with SUDs are compounding given the chronic nature of exposure to substance use, thereby making it difficult to tease apart the individual effects of prenatal exposure from other experiences during childhood.

Case Study 2.1: The Impact of Early Experiences
A 21-year-old female patient named KB is repeatedly getting admitted to a referral psychiatric hospital with a history of being violent towards her family members and threatening to kill anyone who comes close to her. She usually settles down within 2 weeks of admission. Recently, she was consulted by a multidisciplinary team and the following information came forth: KB lost both her parents in a tragic motor vehicle accident at the age of 5 and had to stay with her uncle who sexually assaulted her until the age of 15 when she ran away from home. She resorted to cannabis and later methcathinone to deal with the resultant feelings of emptiness she felt. (K. Molebatsi, personal communication, June 5, 2021).

Stop and Reflect
Discuss with a colleague after reading the case.

1. Identify the adverse childhood experiences in the case.
2. What are the possible differential diagnoses? List points to support each diagnosis.
3. Whose responsibility would it be to manage KB holistically?
4. What preventive measures could be employed to avoid situations such as these?
5. Comment on KB's prognosis.

Effects of parental or caregiver substance use on the family are widespread and may include economic difficulties, forensic or legal matters, unmet developmental needs, family breakdowns, leading to an increased risk of developing emotional, behavioural or substance use problems in children (Alvarez-Monjaras et al., 2019; Barrocas et al., 2016; Rutherford & Mayes, 2017). Attachment theory provides a framework for understanding how SUDs affect the whole family (Bowlby, 1969). A parent/caregiver with a substance use disorder may spend most time intoxicated and/or recovering from the effects of substances at the expense of developing a healthy attachment with their child (Parolin & Simonelli, 2016). Healthy attachment provides protection against psychological problems and illnesses; in its absence a child is more vulnerable to stress and therefore more susceptible to having mental health problems such as SUDs.

Role of Psychological Factors in the Development of SUDs

The interest in personality as a factor in SUDs comes from the observations that despite ACEs and genetic vulnerability, not everyone who is at risk of developing SUDs goes on to do so. Personality is "the enduring configuration of characteristics and behaviour that comprises an individual's unique adjustment to life, including major traits, interests, drives, values, self-concept, abilities, and emotional patterns" (VandenBos, 2007, p. 799). There have been numerous personality characteristics associated with SUDs, including sensation-seeking and impulsivity, although the direction of the relationship is yet to be established. One psychological factor associated with SUDs is motivation. Motivation is "the impetus that gives purpose or direction to behaviour and operates in humans at a conscious or unconscious level" (VandenBos, 2007, p. 687). Studies of motivation in SUDs have focused on providing an explanation of choice, from the reinforcing effects of the 'high' and the avoidance of the negative withdrawal symptoms, to predicting successful completion of rehabilitation treatment and continued abstinence (Goeders, 2004).

Case Study 2.2: JV and SUDs
JV (30 years old) is referred to a rehabilitation centre for further assessment and management. He presented with complaints of stealing, SUD, poor problem solving and attention, poor communication skills, and impulsivity. He started stealing when he was around 11 years old to help meet the needs of his family, who could not afford necessities. He has continued to steal to be able to afford alcohol and khat. According to JV, his parents were very neglectful due to their own struggles with mental illness and substance use. His mother has a history of bipolar disorder and his father has a history of alcohol use disorder. JV reports that often he was left in charge of taking care of his 4 siblings. His father used to come home in a drunken rage and beat his wife and children. JV initially started with smoking cigarettes at 12 because of peer pressure, and started drinking at 15 years old. He dropped out of school at 16. He started using khat 5 years ago when alcohol was no longer as effective at making him 'feel better'.

JV has attempted rehabilitation treatment in the past but finds himself regressing due to painful withdrawal symptoms. His friends describe him as irresponsible and unable to make good decisions even when his choices have poor consequences.
(S. Rampa, personal communication, May 15, 2021)

Stop and Reflect
Discuss the following with a colleague after reading the case:

1. What developmental risk factors can you identify that made JV more vulnerable to developing alcohol and khat use disorders? Be sure to discuss biological, psychological, and social factors.
2. If JV was to undergo neuroimaging assessment, what would the radiologist expect to find in his frontal lobes? Why?
3. How would dopaminergic activity explain JV's struggles with successfully completing rehabilitation treatment?

The relationship between psychological problems and SUDs is bi-directional, in that SUDs are a risk factor for mental illness, but also that self-medication of mental illness is often a reason for continued substance use and SUDs (Volkow, 2004). Substance use is commonly initiated in adolescence or early adulthood and previous research has demonstrated a link between the age of onset of substance use and psychosocial problems. For example, early initiation of substance use is more likely to result in dropping out of school, adjustment problems, and severe psychological problems.

Conclusion

SUDs are multimodal in nature and require a holistic approach to understanding the risk factors that increase a person's vulnerability. Early models of SUDs emphasised individual components; however, they fall short of providing a comprehensive explanation of SUDs. The developmental approach allows for researchers, clinicians, public health specialists, and other relevant stakeholders to have a better picture of the interaction between the different components of an individual's experiences. Furthermore, the disproportionate rates of substance use/misuse during adolescence, compared to other age groups, further illustrates the necessity to address developmental factors. Given the strained resources of sub-Saharan countries, a biopsychosocial approach to addressing the increasing burden caused by SUDs is a positive step towards an integrated framework that targets the key drivers of SUDs.

End of Chapter Questions

1. Which of the models described in this chapter best explain how SUDs are understood in your community?
2. What are the implications of adopting each of the above models when developing and implementing public health policies targeting SUDs?
3. What are the implications of adopting each of the above models when developing and implementing treatments and interventions for SUDs?
4. What are the advantages of adopting a developmental framework for addressing SUDs within your community?
5. What are the challenges of adopting a developmental framework for addressing SUDs within your community?

References

Ajonijebu, D. C., Abboussi, O., Russell, V. A., Mabandla, M. V., & Daniels, W. M. U. (2017). Epigenetics: A link between addiction and social environment. *Cellular and Molecular Life Sciences, 74*(15), 2735–2747. https://doi.org/10.1007/s00018-017-2493-1

Alvarez-Monjaras, M., Mayes, L. C., Potenza, M. N., & Rutherford, H. J. (2019). A developmental model of addictions: Integrating neurobiological and psychodynamic theories through the lens of attachment. *Attachment & Human Development, 21*(6), 616–637. https://doi.org/10/gjkkvw

American Psychiatric Association. (2013). Diagnostic and statistical manual of mental disorders (5th ed.). https://doi.org/10.1176/appi.books.9780890425596

Barrocas, J., Vieira-Santos, S., & Paixão, R. (2016). Parenting and drug addiction: A psychodynamic proposal based on a multifactorial perspective. *Psychoanalytic Psychology, 33*(1), 161–178. https://doi.org/10/f79z23

Bowlby, J. (1969). *Attachment and loss.* Basic Books.

Caritis, S. N., & Panigrahy, A. (2019). Opioids affect the fetal brain: Reframing the detoxification debate. *American Journal of Obstetrics and Gynecology, 221*(6), 602–608. https://doi.org/10/gjpmq6

Carlier, J., Huestis, M. A., Zaami, S., Pichini, S., & Busardò, F. P. (2020). Monitoring perinatal exposure to cannabis and synthetic cannabinoids. *Therapeutic Drug Monitoring, 42*(2), 194–204. https://doi.org/10/ggfck3

Chambers, R. A., Taylor, J. R., & Potenza, M. N. (2003). Developmental neurocircuitry of motivation in adolescence: A critical period of addiction vulnerability. *American Journal of Psychiatry, 160*(6), 1041–1052. https://doi.org/10.1176/appi.ajp.160.6.1041

Cicchetti, D., & Handley, E. D. (2019). Child maltreatment and the development of substance use and disorder. *Neurobiology of Stress, 10*, 100144. https://doi.org/10.1016/j.ynstr.2018.100144

DeMartino, C. H., Rice, R. E., & Saltz, R. (2015). An applied test of the social learning theory of deviance to college alcohol use. *Journal of Health Communication, 20*(4), 479–490. https://doi.org/10/gf9mnj

Feltenstein, M. W., & See, R. E. (2008). The neurocircuitry of addiction: An overview. *British Journal of Pharmacology, 154*(2), 261–274. https://doi.org/10.1038/bjp.2008.51

Frank, L. E., & Nagel, S. K. (2017). Addiction and moralization: The role of the underlying model of addiction. *Neuroethics, 10*(1), 129–139. https://doi.org/10/gbjd6b

Goeders, N. E. (2004). Stress, motivation, and drug addiction. *Current Directions in Psychological Science, 13*(1), 33–35. https://doi.org/10/bdr99j

Hall, W., Carter, A., & Barnett, A. (2017). Disease or developmental disorder: Competing perspectives on the neuroscience of addiction. *Neuroethics, 10*(1), 103–110. https://doi.org/10.1007/s12152-017-9303-1

Hamilton, P. J., & Nestler, E. J. (2019). Epigenetics and addiction. *Current Opinion in Neurobiology, 59*, 128–136. https://doi.org/10.1016/j.conb.2019.05.005

Heather, N. (2017). Q: Is addiction a brain disease or a moral failing? A: Neither. *Neuroethics, 10*(1), 115–124. https://doi.org/10/gjkkwh

Kabiru, C. W., Beguy, D., Crichton, J., & Ezeh, A. C. (2010). Self-reported drunkenness among adolescents in four sub-Saharan African countries: Associations with adverse childhood experiences. *Child and Adolescent Psychiatry and Mental Health, 4*(1), 17. https://doi.org/10.1186/1753-2000-4-17

Kiburi, S. K., Molebatsi, K., Obondo, A., & Kuria, M. W. (2018). Adverse childhood experiences among patients with substance use disorders at a referral psychiatric hospital in Kenya. *BMC Psychiatry, 18*(1), 197. https://doi.org/10.1186/s12888-018-1780-1

Koob, G. F. (2009). Brain stress systems in the amygdala and addiction. *Brain Research, 1293*, 61–75. https://doi.org/10/crjv3m

Koob, G. F. (2017). Antireward, compulsivity, and addiction: Seminal contributions of Dr. Athina Markou to motivational dysregulation in addiction. *Psychopharmacology, 234*(9–10), 1315–1332. https://doi.org/10/f972z5

Krohn, M. D., Skinner, W. F., Massey, J. L., & Akers, R. L. (1985). Social learning theory and adolescent cigarette smoking: A longitudinal study. *Social Problems, 32*(5), 455–473. https://doi.org/10/gjnrtv

Kruis, N. E., Seo, C., & Kim, B. (2020). Revisiting the empirical status of social learning theory on substance use: A systematic review and meta-analysis. *Substance Use & Misuse, 55*(4), 666–683. https://doi.org/10/gjnrw7

Love, B., Vetere, A., & Davis, P. (2020). Understanding addiction, relapse and recovery amongst substance using offenders – A qualitative study informed by developmental psychological theories. *Drugs and Alcohol Today, 20*(4), 337–352. https://doi.org/10.1108/DAT-04-2020-0023.

Mattson, S. N., Bernes, G. A., & Doyle, L. R. (2019). Fetal alcohol spectrum disorders: A review of the neurobehavioral deficits associated with prenatal alcohol exposure. *Alcoholism: Clinical and Experimental Research, 43*(6), 1046–1062.

McCrory, E. J., & Mayes, L. (2015). Understanding addiction as a developmental disorder: An argument for a developmentally informed multilevel approach. *Current Addiction Reports, 2*(4), 326–330. https://doi.org/10.1007/s40429-015-0079-2.

Niaura, R. (2000). Cognitive social learning and related perspectives on drug craving. *Addiction, 95*(8s2), 155–163. https://doi.org/10/ffnb7n.

Oladeji, B. D., Makanjuola, V. A., & Gureje, O. (2010). Family-related adverse childhood experiences as risk factors for psychiatric disorders in Nigeria. *British Journal of Psychiatry, 196*(3), 186–191. https://doi.org/10.1192/bjp.bp.109.063677.

Parolin, M., & Simonelli, A. (2016). Attachment theory and maternal drug addiction: The contribution to parenting interventions. *Frontiers in Psychiatry, 7*. https://doi.org/10/gjs7f7

Pickard, H. (2020). What we're not talking about when we talk about addiction. *Hastings Center Report, 50*(4), 37–46. https://doi.org/10.1002/hast.1172.

Pierce, R. C., Fant, B., Swinford-Jackson, S. E., Heller, E. A., Berrettini, W. H., & Wimmer, M. E. (2018). Environmental, genetic and epigenetic contributions to cocaine addiction. *Neuropsychopharmacology, 43*(7), 1471–1480. https://doi.org/10.1038/s41386-018-0008-x.

Rutherford, H. J., & Mayes, L. C. (2017). Parenting and addiction: Neurobiological insights. *Current Opinion in Psychology, 15*, 55–60. https://doi.org/10.1016/j.copsyc.2017.02.014.

Schempf, A. H. (2007). Illicit drug use and neonatal outcomes: A critical review. *Obstetrical & Gynecological Survey, 62*(11), 749–757. https://doi.org/10/cqnnk3

See, R. E., Fuchs, R. A., Ledford, C. C., & McLaughlin, J. (2003). Drug addiction, relapse, and the amygdala. *Annals of the New York Academy of Sciences, 985*(1), 294–307. https://doi.org/10/b5v7md

Sherr, L., Croome, N., Bradshaw, K., & Parra Castaneda, K. (2014). A systematic review examining whether interventions are effective in reducing cognitive delay in children infected and affected with HIV. *AIDS Care, 26*(Suppl 1), S70–S77. https://doi.org/10.1080/09540121.2014.906560.

Smith, V. C., Wilson, C. R., & Prevention, C. on S.U.A. (2016). Families affected by parental substance use. *Pediatrics, 138*(2) https://doi.org/10.1542/peds.2016-1575.

Stockdale, S. E., Wells, K. B., Tang, L., Belin, T. R., Zhang, L., & Sherbourne, C. D. (2007). The importance of social context: Neighborhood stressors, stress-buffering mechanisms, and alcohol, drug, and mental health disorders. *Social Science and Medicine, 65*(9), 1867–1881. https://doi.org/10.1016/j.socscimed.2007.05.045.

VandenBos, G. R. (2007). *APA dictionary of psychology*. American Psychological Association.

Volkow, N., Koob, G. F., & McLellan, A. T. (2016). Neurobiologic advances from the brain disease model of addiction. *New England Journal of Medicine, 374*(4), 363–371. https://doi.org/10/gcwbv4

Volkow, N., & Li, T.-K. (2005). The neuroscience of addiction. *Nature Neuroscience, 8*(11), 1429–1430. https://doi.org/10.1038/nn1105-1429.

Volkow, N., & Muenke, M. (2012). The genetics of addiction. *Human Genetics, 131*(6), 773–777. https://doi.org/10.1007/s00439-012-1173-3

Volkow, N. D. (2004). The reality of comorbidity: Depression and drug abuse. *Biological Psychiatry, 56*(10), 714–717. https://doi.org/10/fngbv4

Whiteman, V. E., Salemi, J. L., Mogos, M. F., Cain, M. A., Aliyu, M. H., & Salihu, H. M. (2014). Maternal opioid drug use during pregnancy and its impact on perinatal morbidity, mortality, and the costs of medical care in the United States. *Journal of Pregnancy, 2014*, e906723. https://doi.org/10/f6r9bn

Wilson, G. T. (1987). Cognitive processes in addiction. *British Journal of Addiction, 82*(4), 343–353. https://doi.org/10/b6v8j9

Wilson, G. T. (1988). Alcohol use and abuse: A social learning analysis. In C. D. Chaudron & D. A. Wilkinson (Eds.), *Theories on alcoholism* (pp. 239–287). Addiction Research Foundation.

CHAPTER 3

Alcohol Use in Sub-Saharan Africa

Philip Opondo, James Ayugi, Anthony Olashore, and Tshephiso Teseletso

Abstract Alcohol is the most widely used and misused substance in sub-Saharan Africa. Globally, 3 million deaths occur annually from harmful use of alcohol, representing 5.3% of all deaths. The World Health Organization (WHO) attributes 5.1% of the global burden of disease and injury to alcohol, measured in disability-adjusted life years (DALYs). Beyond health consequences, the harmful use of alcohol leads to significant socio-economic losses to individuals, families, and communities. This chapter explores various aspects related to the use of alcohol, current alcohol consumption patterns in sub-Saharan Africa and elsewhere, as well as the related burden of diseases attributable to its harmful use. Theoretical models underpinning the disease model of alcohol use and misuse together with the current

P. Opondo (✉) • J. Ayugi • A. Olashore
University of Botswana, Gaborone, Botswana

Sbrana Hospital, Lobatse, Botswana
e-mail: Opondopr@ub.ac.bw; ayugij@ub.ac.bw; olashorea@ub.ac.bw

T. Teseletso
Gaborone Rehabilitation and Emergency Centre, Gaborone, Botswana

M. Mhaka-Mutepfa (ed.), *Substance Use and Misuse in sub-Saharan Africa*, https://doi.org/10.1007/978-3-030-85732-5_3

understanding on aetiological and risk factors are discussed. The chapter concludes by discussing the challenges and opportunities in tackling alcohol use disorder in local contexts and offers suggestions for interventions.

Keywords Alcohol use/misuse • Risk factors • Socio-economic losses • Injuries • Behavioural and mental disorders • Health consequences • Interventions

Introduction

Given the abundant raw materials for production, alcohol has always been easily available, and forms a fundamental and indispensable part of traditional African culture. It was largely consumed for social occasions such as weddings, cultural festivals, and rituals (see Lyumugabe et al., 2010). However, alcohol consumption has increased (Wilsnack et al., 2005) and this could explain the increase in the prevalence of alcohol misuse and alcohol dependence in sub-Saharan Africa in recent years. The Diagnostic and Statistical Manual of Mental Disorders (DSM 5) combined alcohol misuse and alcohol dependence into one disorder: alcohol use disorder (AUD) (American Psychiatric Association [APA], 2013). AUD is a challenging pattern of alcohol misuse that leads to distress and impairment in functioning (APA, 2013). It is a condition that arises out of and is maintained by several social, psychological, neurobiological, and external risk factors. The risk factors may interact in diverse ways to trigger the development of AUD. The psychosocial factors influencing alcohol use found in previous studies comprise peer influence, stress, religious beliefs, several demographics, and personality traits among others (Ndetei et al., 2009; Olashore et al., 2018). Biological factors include genetic factors, sex, and metabolic variations. Environmental factors comprise ease of access and the nature of the home and social environment. The causes and risk factors are discussed below. However, readers should note that since the causes for excessive alcohol use are similar to those of other substances, aetiology covers the different types of substances.

Social Factors Leading to Substance Use Including Alcohol

As suggested by Olashore et al. (2018), several aspects in the life of users have a bearing on their vulnerability to use substances. Early childhood experiences (ECE) have the capacity to either diminish or enhance the potential of a young adolescent to use substances later on in life. (Tapera et al., 2020). For instance, some young people are from backgrounds that are chaotic, a phenomenon which puts them at an increased risk for using substances (Moitlakgola & Amone-P'Olak, 2015). The aforementioned authors posited that adverse childhood experiences (ACEs) have been documented to influence substance use amongst young people and carrying on into adulthood. ACEs include, among others, childhood neglect, child sexual abuse, witnessing domestic violence acts and exposure to family members who were using substances. In trying to deal with such circumstances, an adolescent may start the use of substances earlier and may also use substances later in life from social learning, encouraging a cycle of intergenerational alcohol misuse and its allied unhealthy family and lifestyle coping patterns.

Another factor is the availability or easy access to substances by young people. Schupmann et al. (2018) reported that school-going adolescents got hooked on substances because of availability at home and at school. Easy access makes the youth with such affinity 3.5 times more likely to use substances later on in life (Riva et al., 2018). In African contexts, access is possible as some homesteads sell traditional beer and children are exposed to it at a young age (see Schupmann et al., 2018). Relatedly, peer pressure has for a long time been an associated risk for drug use and is instrumental in making adolescents use substances (Jaccard et al., 2005; Tapera et al., 2020; Mbongwe et al., 2018). Adolescents with friends who use substances are more likely to use substances themselves.

Case Study 3.1: I Am Never Enough, Not Man Enough for him
Z was an obedient, humble 19-year-old pursuing medicine in a prestigious university but succumbed to peer pressure. Each time he felt under pressure and tried to talk with his father, the father would say "You are weak and useless". His mother was a submissive cultured woman who couldn't confront the father but quietly encouraged her son to ignore his father's remarks. However, Z's grades dropped, and he lost interest in his studies. He came home often smelling of alcohol and talked of pursuing a football and Disk Jockey career. His father threatened to disown him. Z's alcohol use increased. They eventually, ended up in therapy and Z said to his father, "...when I was 7, I scored that penalty and you said it was a stroke of luck; the feeling of my inadequacy is always reflected in your eyes and words...it's one of the saddest things that make me want to stay away from home and be with my friends instead'. Z's father laughed out loud and responded, "For the first time ever be a man and don't embarrass me in front of the psychologist". (T. Teseletso, personal communication, November 20, 2020)

Stop and Reflect

1. Explore the role of upbringing and its influence on alcohol use in this case.
2. What should be the attitude of parents towards children?
3. Should more be done for the boy-child regarding the societal expectations placed upon them?
4. What would be your role in helping Student Z and his family? Explain how you will help each family member.

Psychological Factors Leading to Substance Use Including Alcohol

Psychological variables can hugely influence and accentuate the use of substances especially amongst the youth. Researchers in Botswana (e.g., Ludick & Amone-P'Olak, 2016) revealed that youth who are excitable and impulsive were more likely to use cannabis. Additionally, Fraser and Plattner (2018) also noted that students with high self-control were able to easily stop drug use, implying that lack of self-control is a risk factor to substance use. Students with self-esteem issues were also found to contemplate substance use (Gareikitse & Plattner, 2016).

Biological Factors Leading to Substance Use Including Alcohol

Genetic factors are strongly implicated in the susceptibility to develop syndromes such as attention-deficit/hyperactivity disorder (ADHD), conduct disorder, and substance use disorders (SUDs) (Iob et al., 2021). Genetic variables have been seen to contribute immensely to use of substances amongst the youth. In a United Kingdom based study, Iob et al. (2021) indicated that the debut of substance use may stem from mental health vulnerabilities and traits that are genetically influenced. For example, a student whose relatives smoke and has negligent parents may also begin smoking or it can be an interaction between environmental exposure and genes. Strong evidence from family, twin, and genome-wide linkage and association studies suggests that genetic factors play a crucial role in shaping the vulnerability to SUDs (Arcos-Burgos et al., 2019) including AUD.

Signs and Symptoms of Alcohol Use Disorder

Many people with AUD will deny having a problem. However, there are several physical, behavioural, and psychological signs and symptoms that can help make a diagnosis. Behavioural signs include neglect of school or work and other social responsibilities (American Psychiatric Association, 2013) as well as aggressive and violent acts (World Health Organization, 2018). AUD can also be indicated by physical withdrawal symptoms including nausea and vomiting, palpitations, hand tremors, sweating and psychological withdrawal symptoms such as sleep problems, hallucinations, and anxiety among others (American Psychiatric Association, 2013). According to the APA (American Psychiatric Association, 2013), in order to be diagnosed with AUD, an individual would have to present with at least 2 out of 11 signs and symptoms including the aforementioned symptoms.

Case Study 3.2: Drinking Gone Awry

Dr X, a 53-year-old surgeon, was involved in a road accident and smelt heavily of alcohol and spoke with a slow slurred speech. Three days after admission he became confused, restless, combative, and he had hallucinations. Dr X had started drinking while in college. He started with one or two beers with friends during weekends and kept increasing the number of beers until he moved to strong stuff after graduating. After marrying, he had frequent fights with his wife after drinking. He also had problems at work due to lateness or absenteeism after drinking bouts. He later developed tremors and could only steady his hands for an operation after taking a swig from the small whisky bottles he carried in his pockets. He had also developed hypertension and diabetes. His wife had threatened to leave him over his drinking and asked him to seek help, but he had adamantly refused saying he had no drinking problem.(J. Ayugi, personal communication, May 5, 2021)

Stop and Reflect

- Is this an alcohol problem or an AUD? Why?
- Discuss intimate partner violence after alcohol use in your communities.
- Why is intimate partner violence prevalent among alcohol users?

Epidemiology of Alcohol Use Disorder

The consumption of alcohol varies across sub-Saharan African countries ranging from less than a litre to more than 10 litres per capita (Obot, 2006). Several indicators can be used to measure the level of alcohol consumption in a country or region (World Health Organization, 2018). These include:

- total alcohol per capita consumption in litres of pure alcohol per person per year
- alcohol consumption in grams of pure alcohol per person per day.

In Africa, the WHO Eastern Mediterranean Region (EMRO), consisting of the Muslim countries in the Middle East and North Africa, has the lowest alcohol consumption in the world, both in terms of total adult per capita consumption (APC) (0.65 litres) and prevalence of non-drinkers, (87.8%) (WHO, 2018). Consumption in the rest of the African region is at an APC of 6.15 and 57.2% of the population are lifetime abstainers (WHO, 2018). Thus, overall, the proportion of the drinking population in Africa is relatively low, while the overall consumption per capita is relatively high.

Binge drinking is common in Africa (Obot, 2006) and globally the highest rate of heavy episodic consumption is found among men and women in sub-Saharan Africa (WHO, 2018). The drinking pattern is important as it may have an association with the complications that develop from alcohol use (Wetterling et al., 1999). Excessive alcohol intake has been well known as the leading risk factor for mortality, morbidity, disability, and disability-adjusted life years (DALYs) among young African males in sub-Saharan Africa aged 15–24 years (Ferreira-Borges et al., 2017). It has also been documented that the prevalence of AUD (defined by an Alcohol Use Disorders Identification Test (AUDIT) score ≥8) is estimated at 3% in Africa (Ferreira-Borges et al., 2017). WHO reported that alcohol causes about 271,000 premature deaths in Africa annually (World Health Organization, 2013).

Alcohol consumption figures differ from one study to another; 81% of African women testified they were non-users, and those who used ranged from 1% (Malawi) to 30% (Burkina Faso). Heavy drinking among users is wide-ranging from 4% (Ghana) to 41% (Chad), and dangerous single-occasion consumption fluctuated from less than 1% (Mauritius) to 58% (Chad) (Martinez et al., 2011). Incidence of alcohol use among women in a previous year was projected at 30% in Botswana and 47% in Namibia (Weiser et al., 2006), which was high despite non-acceptance of female drinking in African cultures, likely due to religion, customs and tradition, and gender roles (Wilsnack et al., 2005). However, this view is changing in some sectors due to acculturation (personal communication, May 2020). In fact, Ferreira-Borges et al. (2015) examined alcohol consumption within sub-Saharan African nations and noted increases in alcohol consumption among women and the youth, with sporadic binge drinking reported the most (Martinez et al., 2011).

Alcohol and Youth

There has been an increase in drinking among the youth. An estimated 43% of those aged 15 years or above have used alcohol before and 30% used it in the previous year (World Health Organization, 2014). In Tanzania, Francis et al. (2015) evaluated alcohol use amongst northern Tanzania youth. This study revealed a significant drinking problem amongst youths (15–24 years) with 71% of males reporting heavy episodic drinking as compared to 27% amongst females. Similar findings of youths drinking more in Botswana were reported (Olashore et al., 2018).

While research is still exploring the reasons for the increasing alcohol use among youth across several countries in sub-Saharan Africa, several potential reasons have been raised including new aggressive marketing strategies by the alcohol industry (De Bruijin et al., 2014), which will be discussed in the next chapter.

Harmful Consequences of Alcohol Misuse

Alcohol misuse has been linked to a host of other deleterious effects and it can virtually affect all organs and systems in the body (American Psychiatric Association, 2013). The harmful use of alcohol is a causal factor associated with many diseases and injury conditions including cardiovascular diseases, diabetes, cancers of the mouth, throat, oesophagus, and liver amongst others (see WHO, 2018) and neuropsychiatric conditions like Wernicke's encephalopathy and alcoholic cerebellar degeneration (Hammoud & Jimenez-Shahad, 2019). Furthermore, excessive use of alcohol has been associated with mental health conditions like depression (WHO, 2018) and suicidality (APA, 2013).

Alcohol and HIV

Alcohol use continues to have a significant impact on the HIV epidemic through multiple pathways including increased sexual risk-taking (Rehm et al., 2017), decreased self-care behaviours such as access to HIV services (Gari et al., 2013), and non-adherence to treatment. Fisher et al. (2007) found that alcohol users were twice as likely to have HIV infection. Alcohol users were also more likely to show faster disease progression, and AUD is more common among people living with HIV than among the general population for they may be trying to cope by resorting to drinking (Kalichman et al., 2007).

High-risk drinking patterns, especially binge drinking, may play an intermediate role between alcohol use and HIV acquisition, and are linked to several non-communicable diseases such as diabetes and hypertension (Francis et al., 2015). This has a large impact on the burden of disease and mortality especially as sub-Saharan Africa has some of the highest HIV prevalence rates globally (UNAIDS, 2021) and high levels of harmful use of alcohol (WHO, 2018).

Social Complications

Alcohol misuse gives rise to a multitude of social problems. These include intimate partner violence, accidents at home, work and road traffic accidents, injuries from fights and brawls, crime, work related problems, and poverty ((Hatcher et al., 2014). Alcohol consumption, especially at harmful and hazardous levels, is a major contributor to the occurrence of intimate partner violence. In South Africa, 65% of women experiencing spousal abuse within the last 12 months reported that their partner always or sometimes used alcohol before the assault (Hatcher et al., 2014). Alcohol use can also lead to disruption of families. The function of a family as a system is to provide shelter as well as emotional, economic, and psychological support; but when one member misuses alcohol, the family becomes destabilized (Schafer, 2011). Money that could have been used for the family is misused on alcohol and this could further contribute to social ills.

Case Study 3.3: I Lost My Family and Now My Job Is on the Line Too

Patient Y had a prestigious job and title with all benefits. Y had a chronic alcohol misuse lifestyle and anger management issues. He was raised by his grandmother. During one family vacation; Y had consumed a lot of alcohol and started to have an uncontrolled argument with his wife and three children, which ended in an almost fatal car accident, leaving the wife with long-term injuries. Patient Y's wife filed for divorce after her recovery. Y was also on the verge of losing his job. (T. Teseletso, personal communication, January 10, 2021)

Stop and Reflect

1. What major social issues need to be addressed with Patient Y?
2. What minor or 'easy to overlook' social factors should be addressed with Patient Y?
3. What social complications have resulted from Patient Y's alcohol misuse?

Social complications of alcohol use can be illuminated by the latest findings on the effects of lack of access to alcohol in South Africa. Lack of access to alcohol led to a colossal drop in unnatural deaths in the country from 800–1000/week to around 400/week during the COVID-19 lockdowns. Patient statistics for assault also fell (from 145 to 64: 55.8%), so did patient figures from accidents (from 207 to 83: 59.9%), patient numbers from other injuries (from 463 to 188:59.4%) and patient figures from sexual assault (from 12 to 1: 91.6%) during the first 2 weeks of lockdown (Morojele et al., 2021). This helped free health services for COVID-19 patients. The significant drop in accident, injury, and assault numbers speak to the harmful effects of alcohol.

Mental Health Complications

Alcohol can affect the brain directly leading to alteration in brain functioning, therefore inducing psychological symptoms (Koob, 2013). Underlying mental health problems may also lead to heavy drinking and complicate the existing psychological issues. AUD may co-exist independently with a mental illness necessitating a dual mental health diagnosis. Therefore, determining the relationship between alcohol use problems and mental health disorders is essential for proper treatment planning and implementation.

The Concept of Alcohol Use Disorders (AUD)

AUD has been conceptualized as a disease for over 200 years and is viewed as a chronic disease (White et al., 2002). Theoretical models that have been used to investigate and explain alcohol use include the Theory of Planned Behavior (see Collins & Carey, 2008) and the Health Belief Model (see Abercromby et al., 2021). The 'kindling'/stress hypothesis also forms a conceptual basis for the development and maintenance of alcohol misuse. Studies done regarding this hypothesis have indicated that repeated withdrawals from chronic low levels of alcohol ignite anxiety-like behaviour, motivating and perpetuating alcohol use (Breese et al., 2005). Another conceptual framework looks at alcoholism as a reward-deficit disorder (Koob, 2013). According to this model, alcoholism affects several motivational dimensions and can be conceptualized as a disorder comprising of a continuum from impulsivity (positive reinforcement) to compulsivity (negative reinforcement). The compulsive drug-seeking reward linked with alcoholism can be mined from multiple neuroadaptations. Through this model of alcohol misuse, the negative emotional state that drives the motivation for negative reinforcement is believed to be due to a dysregulation of specific neurochemical elements involved in reward and stress in the basal forebrain structures, namely the ventral striatum and extended amygdala (Koob, 2013).

Treatment of Alcohol Use Disorder

Many people who have AUD in low- and middle-income countries, especially in sub-Saharan Africa, do not get treated and the few who get treated usually do so in the late stages when complications have arisen (Benegal et al., 2009). There are, however, treatment options available and they are briefly discussed in this chapter as Chaps. 10 and 11 cover prevention and intervention in cases of substance use, inclusive of alcohol.

Brief Interventions

Initial screening for alcohol use problems can be effectively carried out in primary care settings using the following tests: Alcohol Use Disorders Identification Test (AUDIT) and Alcohol, Smoking and Substance Involvement Screening Test (ASSIST) (see Chap. 11). Interventions in primary health care institutions following screening are very often effective in reducing alcohol consumption (Sullivan et al., 2011).

Psychological and Pharmacological Interventions

Psychological interventions including crisis intervention, motivational interviewing, and cognitive behavioural therapy are used in the treatment of AUD and will be discussed in detail in Chap. 11. However, the management of AUD involves both psychosocial approaches and the use of adjunctive medications. The most used medications have been naltrexone, acamprosate, and disulfiram. Other medications used are anticonvulsants and antidepressants which are used off-label. Disulfiram acts by inhibiting the enzyme aldehyde dehydrogenase which is involved in the metabolism of alcohol. Naltrexone is an opioid antagonist while acamprosate is an N-methyl- D-aspartate (NMDA) receptor blocker. Most of these medications may not be available in primary care centres in sub-Saharan Africa; their use is therefore mostly initiated by specialists.

Management of Alcohol Withdrawal

For patients with AUD, benzodiazepines are used as first-line medication for the management of alcohol withdrawal. Antipsychotic medications can be added as adjunct treatment when indicated. Oral or intravenous/intramuscular thiamine is used when there is evidence of Wernicke's encephalopathy or severe malnutrition. To prevent relapse in alcohol dependent patients, medical doctors prescribe acamprosate, disulfiram, or naltrexone depending on patient preference. Psychologists provide psychosocial support for patients with AUD and where possible, provide or refer for more structured therapies and provision for family support. Stakeholders should encourage utilization of self-help groups such as Alcoholics Anonymous (AA) where available. Other groups like Narcotics Anonymous or religious-based 12-Step groups have adopted the AA model to deal with substance issues (see Donovan et al., 2013).

Conclusion

End of Chapter Questions

1. Why are there gender differences in alcohol consumption from a cultural point of view?
2. Why are prevalence rates significantly different across countries? Discuss.
3. Why are alcohol consumption rates among women rising? Discuss.
4. Discuss and write a group assignment of what transpires during AA and the steps followed to make them effective.
5. Choose any relevant theory and use it to explain alcohol use disorder.
6. What should institutions do to reduce alcohol misuse patterns in sub-Saharan Africa?
7. What could you do differently to build a more effective response to the heavy episodic drinking in sub-Saharan Africa?
8. Which theorist would make better explanation of the interplay of adverse childhood experiences and the initiation of substance use, what would they say, and why?

References

Abercromby, M., Leavy, J. E., Tohotoa, J., Bona, M. D., Nimmo, L., & Crawford, G. (2021). "Go hard or go home": Exploring young people's knowledge, attitudes and behaviours of alcohol use and water safety in Western Australia using the health belief model. *International Journal of Health Promotion and Education, 59*(3), 174–191. https://doi.org/10.1080/14635240.2020.1759441.

American Psychiatric Association. (2013). *Diagnostic and statistical manual of mental disorders* (5th ed.). American Psychiatric Association.

Amone-P'Olak, K., Chilunga, W., Omech, B., & Opondo, P. R. (2020). Knowledge of alcohol-disease links and socio-demographic factors as predictors of support for alcohol-related policies among university students in Botswana. *Drugs: Education, Prevention & Policy, 27*(4), 320–327. https://doi.org/10.1080/09687637.2019.1664994.

Arcos-Burgos, M., Vélez, J. I., … Martinez, A. F. (2019). ADGRL3 (LPHN3) variants predict substance use disorder. *Translational Psychiatry, 9*(42) https://doi.org/10.1038/s41398-019-0396-7.

Benegal, V., Chand, P. K., & Obot, I. S. (2009). Packages of care for alcohol use disorders in low-and middle-income countries. *PLoS Medicine, 6*(10), 1–7. e1000170.

Breese, G., Overstreet, D., & Knapp, D. (2005). Conceptual framework for the etiology of alcoholism: A "kindling" /stress hypothesis. *Psychopharmacology, 178*, 367–380. https://doi.org/10.1007/s00213-004-2016-2.

Collins, S. E., & Carey, K. (2008). The theory of planned behavior as a model of heavy episodic drinking among college students. *Psychology of Addictive Behaviours, 21*(4), 498–507. https://doi.org/10.1037/0893-164X.21.4.498.

De Bruijin, A., Ferreira-Borges, C., Engels, R., & Bhavsar, M. (2014). Monitoring outdoor alcohol advertising in developing countries: Findings of a pilot study in five African countries. *African Journal of Drug and Alcohol Studies, 13*(1), 12–29.

Donovan, D. M., Ingalsbe, M. H., Benbow, J., & Daley, D. C. (2013). 12-step interventions and mutual support programs for substance use disorders: An overview. *Social Work in Public Health, 28*(3–4), 313–332. https://doi.org/10.1080/19371918.2013.774663.

Ferreira-Borges, C., Esser, M. B., Dias, S., Babor, T., & Parry, C. D. (2015). Alcohol control policies in 46 African countries: Opportunities for improvement. *Alcohol and Alcoholism, 50*(4), 470–476.

Ferreira-Borges, C., Parry, C. D., & Babor, T. F. (2017). Harmful use of alcohol: A shadow over sub-Saharan Africa in need of workable solutions. *International Journal of Environmental Research and Public Health, 14*(4), 346.

Fisher, J. C., Bang, H., & Kapiga, S. H. (2007). The association between HIV infection and alcohol use: A systematic review and meta-analysis of African studies. *Sexually Transmitted Diseases, 34*(11), 856–863.

Francis, J. M., Weiss, H. A., Mshana, G., Baisley, K., Grosskurth, H., & Kapiga, S. H. (2015). The epidemiology of alcohol use and alcohol use disorders among young people in northern Tanzania. *PLoS One, 10*(10), 1–17. e0140041.

Fraser, L. N., & Plattner, I. E. (2018). Self-control as a predictor of drug use: A study with university students in Botswana. *African Journal of Drug and Alcohol Studies, 17*(1), 30–38.

Gareikitse, M., & Plattner, I. E. (2016). Self-esteem and alcohol dependence as predictors of contemplation to use drugs among university students in Botswana. *African Journal of Drug & Alcohol Studies, 15*(1), 38–47.

Gari, S., Doig-Acuña, C., Smail, T., Malungo, J. R., Martin-Hilber, A., & Merten, S. (2013). Access to HIV/AIDS care: A systematic review of socio-cultural determinants in low and high income countries. *BMC Health Services Research, 13*(1), 1–13.

Griswold, M. G., Fullman, N., Hawley, C., Arian, N., Zimsen, S. R., Tymeson, H. D., … Salama, J. S. (2018). Alcohol use and burden for 195 countries and territories, 1990–2016: A systematic analysis for the global burden of disease study 2016. *The Lancet, 392*, 1015–1035.

Hammoud, N., & Jimenez-Shahad, J. (2019). Chronic neurologic effects of alcohol. *Clinics in Liver Disease, 23*(1), 141–155. https://doi.org/10.1016/j.cld.2018.09.010.

Hatcher, A. M., Colvin, C. J., Ndlovu, N., & Dworkin, S. L. (2014). Intimate partner violence among rural South African men: Alcohol use, sexual decision-making, and partner communication. *Culture, Health & Sexuality, 16*(9), 1023–1039.

Iob, E., Schoeler, T., Cecil, C. M., Walton, E., McQuillin, A., & Pingault, J. (2021). Identifying risk factors involved in the common versus specific liabilities to substance use: A genetically informed approach. *Addiction Biology, 26*(3) https://doi.org/10.1111/adb.12944.

Jaccard, J., Blanton, H., & Dodge, T. (2005). Peer influences on risk behavior: An analysis of the effects of a close friend. *Developmental Psychology, 41*(1), 135–147. https://doi.org/10.1037/0012-1649.

Kalichman, S. C., Simbayi, L. C., Kaufman, M., Cain, D., & Jooste, S. (2007). Alcohol use and sexual risks for HIV/AIDS in sub-Saharan Africa: Systematic review of empirical findings. *Prevention Science, 8*(2), 141–151.

Koob, G. F. (2013). Theoretical frameworks and mechanistic aspects of alcohol addiction: Alcohol addiction as a reward deficit disorder. *Current Topics in Behavioural Neuroscience, 13*, 3–30. https://doi.org/10.1007/7854_2011_129.

Ludick, W. K., & Amone-P'Olak, K. (2016). Temperament and the risk of alcohol, tobacco, and cannabis use among university students in Botswana. *African Journal of Drug and Alcohol Studies, 15*(1), 21–35.

Lyumugabe, F., Kamaliza, G., Bajyana, E., & Thonart, P. (2010). Microbiological and physico-chemical characteristic of Rwandese traditional beer "Ikigage". *African Journal of Biotechnology, 9*(27), 4241–4246.

Martinez, P., Røislien, J., Naidoo, N., & Clausen, T. (2011). Alcohol abstinence and drinking among African women: Data from the World Health Surveys. *BMC Public Health, 11*(1), 1–9.

Mbongwe, B., Tapera, R., Katlholo, T., Erick, P., Rahube, T., Nsebula, N., Mokgethi, I., Chuma, M., Boitumelo, K., Molebatsi, M., & Tumoyagae, T. (2018). *Situational analysis on tobacco control in Botswana*. University of Botswana. Gaborone, Botswana.

Moitlakgola, K. K., & Amone-P'Olak, K. (2015). Stressful life events and alcohol use among university students in Botswana. *African Journal of Drug and Alcohol Studies, 14*(2), 81–93.

Morojele, N. K., Dumbili, E. W., Obot, I. S., & Parry, C. (2021). Alcohol consumption, harms and policy developments in sub-Saharan Africa: The case for stronger national and regional responses. *Drug and Alcohol Review, 40*(3), 402–419.

Ndetei, D. M., Khasakhala, L. I., Mutiso, V., Ongecha-Owuor, F. A., & Kokonya, D. A. (2009). Psychosocial and health aspects of drug use by students in public secondary schools in Nairobi, Kenya. *Substance Abuse, 30*(1), 61–68.

Obot, I. S. (2006). Alcohol use and related problems in sub-Saharan Africa. *African Journal of Drug and Alcohol Studies, 5*(1), 17–26.

Olashore, A. A., Ogunwobi, O., Totego, E., & Opondo, P. R. (2018). Psychoactive substance use among first-year students in a Botswana University: Pattern and demographic correlates. *BMC Psychiatry, 18*(1), 270.

Rehm, J., Probst, C., Shield, K. D., & Shuper, P. A. (2017). Does alcohol use have a causal effect on HIV incidence and disease progression? A review of the literature and a modeling strategy for quantifying the effect. *Population Health Metrics, 15*(1), 1–7.

Riva, K., Allen-Taylor, L., Schupmann, W. D., Mphele, S., Moshashane, N., & Lowenthal, E. D. (2018). Prevalence and predictors of alcohol and drug use among secondary school students in Botswana: A cross-sectional study. *BMC Public Health, 18*, 1396. https://doi.org/10.1186/s12889-018-6263-2.

Schafer, G. (2011). Family functioning in families with alcohol and other drug addiction. *Social Policy Journal of New Zealand, 37*(2), 135–151.

Schupmann, W., Riva, K., Mphele, S., Moshashane, N., Matesva, M., & Lowenthal, E. (2018). Phenomenology of substance use among school-going adolescents in Botswana. *International Journal of School Health, 5*(4), 1–7. https://doi.org/10.5812/intjsh.82879

Sullivan, L. E., Tetrault, J. M., Braithwaite, R. S., Turner, B. J., & Fiellin, D. A. (2011). A meta-analysis of the efficacy of nonphysician brief interventions for unhealthy alcohol use: Implications for the patient-centered medical home. *The American Journal on Addictions, 20*(4), 343–356.

Swahn, M. H., Ali, B., Palmier, J. B., Sikazwe, G., & Mayeya, J. (2011). Alcohol marketing, drunkenness, and problem drinking among Zambian youth: findings from the 2004 Global School-Based Student Health Survey. *Journal of Environmental and Public Health, 2011*, 1–8.

Tapera R., Mbongwe, B., Mhaka-Mutepfa, M., Lord, A., Phaladze, N. A., & Zetola., N. M. (2020). The theory of planned behavior as a behavior change model for tobacco control strategies among adolescents in Botswana. *PLoS ONE, 15*(6). https://doi.org/10.1371/journal.pone.0233462.

UNAIDS. (2021). *Fact sheet 2021: Preliminary UNAIDS 2021 epidemiological estimates.* UNAIDS. https://aidsinfo.unaids.org

Weiser, S. D., Leiter, K., Heisler, M., McFarland, W., Percy-de Korte, F., DeMonner, S. M., & Bangsberg, D. R. (2006). A population-based study on alcohol and high-risk sexual behaviors in Botswana. *PLoS Medicine, 3*(10), e392.

Wetterling, T., Veltrup, C., Driessen, M., & John, U. (1999). Drinking pattern and alcohol-related medical disorders. *Alcohol and Alcoholism, 34*(3), 330–336.

White, W. L., Boyle, M., & Loveland, D. (2002). Alcoholism/addiction as a chronic disease: From rhetoric to clinical reality. *Alcoholism Treatment Quarterly, 20*(3–4), 107–129.

Wilsnack, R. W., Wilsnack, S. C., & Obot, I. S. (2005). *Why study gender, alcohol and culture? Alcohol, gender and drinking problems: Perspectives from low and middle income countries.* World Health Organization.

World Health Organisation. (2004). *Global status report on alcohol and health, 2004.* World Health Organization.

World Health Organisation. (2013). *Alcohol consumption and harm in the African region: Status report.* World Health Organization.

World Health Organisation. (2014). *Global status report on alcohol and health, 2014.* World Health Organization.

World Health Organisation. (2018). *Global status report on alcohol and health, 2018.* World Health Organization.

CHAPTER 4

Alcohol Policies and the Marketing Strategies of the Alcohol Industry

Kesego Mathoothe, Leonne Mfolwe, and Magen Mhaka-Mutepfa

Abstract The rate of alcohol consumption and its health and socio-economic effects have been discussed in Chap. 3. This chapter presents a summary of the policies (guidelines and laws) that control and mitigate the use of alcohol, using examples from different countries in sub-Saharan Africa. The intensified marketing and policy interference activities by those who produce alcohol, some of which are resisted by private and public

K. Mathoothe (✉)
Department of Public Health Management, Institute of Development Management in Botswana, Gaborone, Botswana

L. Mfolwe
Department of Psychology, Faculty of Social Sciences, University of Botswana, Gaborone, Botswana
e-mail: mfolwel@ub.ac.bw

M. Mhaka-Mutepfa
Department of Psychology, Faculty of Social Sciences, University of Botswana, Gaborone, Botswana
e-mail: mutepfam@ub.ac.bw

M. Mhaka-Mutepfa (ed.), *Substance Use and Misuse in sub-Saharan Africa*, https://doi.org/10.1007/978-3-030-85732-5_4

health advocates, are also discussed. Governments' control measures that aim to counter the alcohol industry interference in policies to reduce alcohol consumption are explored. Best practices on policies that are aimed at resisting pressures from alcohol corporations are discussed. Lastly, a brief discussion on how government commitment is necessary for the effective adoption and implementation of alcohol policies is offered.

Keywords Alcohol policies • Alcohol industry • Marketing strategies • Rules and regulations • Alcohol substance use

Introduction

As discussed in Chap. 3, the harmful use of alcohol is one of the main risk factors for public health and poses serious health, social and economic consequences (World Health Organiztion, 2011). For instance, high HIV prevalence rates, high levels of gender-based violence (GBV), and emerging problems of non-communicable diseases (NCDs) have been noted globally (World Health Organization, 2014). Alcohol misuse is a key determinant of morbidity and mortality, and a leading correlate of road traffic casualties (World Health Organization, 2018). The harmful use of alcohol has become burdensome to the development of affected countries in sub-Saharan Africa and elsewhere, particularly because some of these regions have weak alcohol policies (Morojele et al., 2021). However, there has been evidence that supports the efficacy of policies (U.S. Department of Health and Human Services, 2016). Research has shown that the formulation of policies that articulate stringent measures to the public with regard to alcohol consumption and misuse can derail alcohol-related problems including alcohol-impaired driving (e.g., Anderson et al., 2009; Ferreira-Borges et al., 2015; Xuan et al., 2015).

The changing alcohol environment in sub-Saharan Africa, where more alcohol is consumed leading to negative health and socio-economic effects, suggests the need for stronger alcohol control and capacity-building policies (Ferreira-Borges et al., 2017; Parry et al., 2012). The implementation of policies may help reduce harm among drinkers, as well as safeguard those who abstain from alcohol. The aforementioned have great potential to decrease alcohol-related disease burden in Africa (Rehm et al., 2006). Studies have shown that the most cost-effective ways to reduce alcohol-related harm is to have regulatory control such as making alcohol less available, less acceptable, more expensive, and prohibiting alcohol advertising (Parry et al., 2012; Ramsoomar & Morojele, 2012). Ferreira-Borges et al. (2015, 2017), Morojele et al. (2021) and Staton et al. (2018) postulated that most sub-Saharan African countries were failing to address the impact of alcohol consumption.

Pitso and Obot (2011) also proclaimed that responses to substance use/misuse in most sub-Saharan African countries have also taken the form of policy and programme formulation. Although alcohol control policies have varied in each country (Ferreira-Borges et al., 2015), policies generally provide a framework that supports prevention strategies (see Chaps. 10 and 11) to ensure their effective and successful implementation (Olawole-Isaac et al., 2018). Strategies to reduce alcohol-related burden have the potential of a reduction rate of up to 25% (Rehm et al., 2006), hence the importance of formation of the WHO Global Strategy to Reduce Harmful Use of Alcohol (World Health Organization, 2010) and the Regional Committee of Africa proposed evidence-based strategies (World Health Organization Regional Office for Africa, 2010). The strategy objectives include implementing alcohol control policies, education and health care interventions, and creating surveillance and monitoring systems for production, consumption, and harm (Ferreira-Borges et al., 2013).

National Alcohol Control Policies

National alcohol policies are documents with set attainable objectives, strategies, and targets to reduce alcohol-related harm (World Health Organization, 2010). Muscat and Pike (2012) found that it is common for alcohol policies to be concerned with health because alcohol is regarded as a health issue globally. However, there are social and economic impacts of alcohol (Moss, 2013; Thavorncharoensap et al., 2009; Saxena et al., 2003) that can be considered when implementing these policies. Perhaps as advances are made in alcohol policies, these too can be incorporated. Countries around the globe participated in the WHO Global Survey on Alcohol and Health 2008, following which some devised and others revised national alcohol control policies as an attempt to respond to the harmful use of alcohol. As a reference, some countries used the Global Strategy against Alcohol Use which has ten priority areas (World Health Organization, 2010), to formulate national alcohol policies. The ten key areas have been listed by the WHO and are as follows: '(1). Leadership, awareness and commitment; (2). Health services' response; (3). Community action; (4). Drink-driving policies and countermeasures;

(5). Availability of alcohol; (6). Marketing of alcoholic beverages; (7). Pricing policies; (8). Reducing the negative consequences of drinking and alcohol intoxication; (9). Reducing the public health impact of illicit alcohol and informally produced alcohol and; (10). Monitoring and surveillance' (see World Health Organization, 2010, p.10).

Studies on national alcohol policies in the sub-Saharan African region have been done with Staton et al. (2018) reviewing alcohol policies for 40 countries. They found that most countries had different low policy restrictiveness ranging from 44.1% in Sao Tomé and Principe to 75.0% in Algeria. The huge range (9–75%) in most of the African countries suggests the differences in strength of alcohol control policies (Staton et al., 2018). The authors also revealed that policy restrictiveness scores were negatively correlated with the amount of alcohol consumed per individual per year ($rs = -0.353$, $P = 0.005$).

Countries should have robust policies to address alcohol consumption and alcohol-related harm in the region, and ascertain that the policies are implemented. For instance, the National Alcohol Policy of Botswana adopted the following eight areas for action (see United Nations Development Programme, 2017) ; (1) inter-sectoral collaboration, (2) increasing community action for support, (3) strengthening public education and awareness, (4) reducing health impacts of alcohol use, (5) ensuring public safety and amenity, (6) responsible marketing, (7) addressing illegally and informally produced alcohol and, (8) research, networking, and exchange of information. In general, most national alcohol policies include the domains of pricing, taxation, physical availability, marketing, and drinking and driving countermeasures (Morojele et al., 2021). Similarities in the aforementioned action areas in national alcohol policies from Malawi (WHO, August, 2017), Uganda (Kalema, 2019), and Botswana (United Nations Development Programme, 2017) have been found. The domains included in most of these national alcohol policies are discussed below.

Price and Tax Policies

The pricing and taxation domain targets pricing according to the type of alcoholic beverage, adjusting the tax rates for inflation and alcohol excise taxes (World Health Organization, 2011). An assessment of the price and tax policies showed that increasing alcohol prices leads to reductions in consumption and alcohol-related social and psychological problems, including alcohol-impaired driving (Babor et al., 2010; Elder et al., 2010; Ferreira-Borges et al., 2015; Rabinovich, et al., 2009; Wagenaar et al., 2009; World Health Organization, 2009; Xu & Chaloupka, 2011). For instance, Wagenaar et al. (2010) postulated that doubling alcohol tax significantly reduces mortality, traffic accidents, aggression, and crime. Vandenberg et al. (2019) and Wagenaar et al. (2010) further established that an increase in alcohol taxes not only reduces consumption but could also be a source of revenue for governments which can be used to fund programmes that prevent alcohol-related harm.

While pricing and taxation policies have the most evidence of effectiveness, most countries in sub-Saharan Africa have alcohol excise taxes but they have not yet been fully explored in terms of their public health and revenue generation benefits (Ferreira-Borges et al., 2017). Nigeria and Botswana were two of the countries with a substantial alcohol tax increase. Nigeria had a 60% increase in alcohol taxes (Okwe, 2016) while Botswana stands at 55% (Masupe et al., 2017). The funds generated had no clear outcome or effectiveness of where they were used in Nigeria (Ferreira-Borges et al., 2017). In the case of Botswana, the funds went into public and school education campaigns; advocating for alcohol-free youth activities; supporting the rehabilitation of survivors of alcohol abuse; regulating the advertising of alcohol in sport activities; and any other related activities (United Nations Development Programme, 2017). This is in line with Masupe et al.'s (2017) suggestion that alcohol taxation alone is not enough to reduce alcohol consumption; and the funds collected from these taxes should be allocated to alcohol misuse prevention and treatment. It is worth noting that Botswana appears to be one of the first countries in sub-Saharan Africa that has made vital strides in implementing stringent tax policies to address detrimental consequences of alcohol (Morojele et al., 2021).

Case Study 4.1: Beer Drinking and Tax Levy Policy

In 2008, as part of the tax policy, an alcohol levy (30%) was introduced by the Government of Botswana to address problematic drinking; the expectation was that alcohol abuse numbers would drop in response to the levy. However, a study by (Sebeelo, 2020) was conducted to assess the effect of levies on alcohol consumption. The study revealed that there was resistance from citizens who drank alcohol and they found alternative ways of searching for and drinking alcohol such as visiting shebeens (Sebeelo, 2020).

Stop and Reflect

1. What did you learn from the case study regarding policies?
2. Identify and discuss other policies in other sub-Saharan African countries on alcohol use.
3. If you were a policy maker, which policies (excluding existing ones) would you put in place to manage alcohol use among the youth?

Policies on Physical Availability

Physical availability policies involve placing restrictions on hours and/or days of sales, consumption in public venues, and outlet density of alcohol, as well as minimum legal purchase age, and licensing of production and retail sales (Babor et al., 2010; WHO, 2012). Alcohol-related crimes were reduced significantly in communities that cut down the numbers of alcohol outlets (Xu et al., 2012; Yu et al., 2008). Additionally, reducing the number of days that alcohol is sold also led to less alcohol-related harm (Middleton et al., 2010). This has been reiterated during the COVID-19 pandemic where alcohol outlets were closed and there was a reduction of traffic accidents and reported cases of violence due to heavy drinking (De Jong et al., 2020).

According to WHO (2011), a fair number of African countries regulate the retail sale of alcoholic beverages, varying by beverage type. Furthermore, these countries more commonly had on-premise sale restrictions (e.g., bars, restaurants) than off-premise restrictions (e.g., liquor stores) and had a minimum legal purchase age (Ferreira-Borges et al., 2015). Some examples of policies that limit the availability of alcohol include the traditional beer regulation and the liquor acts (e.g., in Zimbabwe, Botswana, etc.).

Willis (2006) reported that traditional alcoholic beverages have been used in Africa for a long time but their production and sale have not always been regulated. The introduction of the traditional beer regulations can address the illegal brewing of the beers to prevent the increased risk of harm to consumers. The traditional beer regulation removes commercially brewed beers from households to designated areas/selling points (United National Development Programme, 2017). The liquor acts, such as Malawi's Liquor Act of 1979 and South African's Liquor Act of 2003, were developed to regulate the manufacturing and selling of liquor by giving business licenses to do so. Furthermore, they stipulate the permitted times that alcohol can be sold (Matanje Mwagomba et al., 2018; South Africa Department of Trade & Industry, 2016). The 2016 South African Liquor Amendment Bill, closely related to the Liquor Act, aims at increasing the drinking age in South Africa from 18 years to 21 years (Sifile, 2016; South Africa Department of Trade & Industry, 2016).

Policies to Reduce Drinking and Driving

Babor et al. (2010) outlined that drinking and driving countermeasures involve lowering the blood alcohol concentration (BAC), having sobriety checkpoints, and random breath testing. A considerable number of sub-Saharan Africa countries had a legal BAC limit for drivers in the general population of 0.05 g/dl to 0.08 g/dl while some did not have a policy based on BAC limits (see World Health Organization, 2011). However, South Africa has been considering a 0.00 g/dl BAC limit for all drivers (South Africa Department of Transport, 2015). Random breath testing and sobriety checkpoints were also common practices in sub-Saharan Africa (Babor et al., 2010). These two methods are difficult to implement due to shortage of resources and training (African Development Bank Transport and ICT Department, 2013) and corruption.

Case Study 4.2: Police Officers' Corruption at Roadblocks Derails Reduction of Accidents

Efforts to attain and maintain road safety are undermined by widespread corruption among police officers in charge of traffic enforcement. In fact, in South Africa, the highest rate of official corruption is committed by traffic police officers. These police officers accept bribes by traffic offenders who want to avoid heavy fines for offences. Some police officers allegedly try to solicit bribes from motorists as an inducement to refrain from arresting them. Offences by motorists include speeding, driving cars that are not road worthy, and driving under the influence. Following the corrupt exchange, said drivers are permitted to continue driving despite the risk of causing road accidents. Such incidents derail efforts to reduce accidents on the road. Some police officers were reported to also drive under the influence.

Adapted from Arrive Alive (n.d.)

Stop and Reflect

1. What is your opinion on the police who fail to uphold the law?
2. What policies and practices could be implemented to eradicate corruption among traffic police officers?
3. Have you witnessed corruption by motorists and law enforcement on the road? Discuss
4. Why do people drive under the influence of alcohol and ignore road laws?
5. How can we curtail drinking and driving?
6. How can corruption for traffic offenses be reduced in your country?

Policies to Reduce the Marketing of Alcohol

Babor et al. (2010) outlined that policies on marketing are concerned with restricting the marketing exposure of alcohol. According to WHO (2011), many of the member states had no legally binding regulations for alcohol marketing but some had restrictions on alcohol sponsorship and retail sales promotion in order to limit alcohol misuse. This can mean that without binding regulations for marketing, alcohol could continue to be misused. The exposure to marketing of alcohol and alcohol misuse has been found to be highly correlated especially among the youths (Swahn et al., 2011). For instance, in Zambia, students aged 11–16 years who had received a free alcoholic beverage from a company representative had significantly high odds of experiencing alcohol use disorders and related problems, like absconding from school or aggression, unlike their counterparts (Swahn et al., 2011). The numbers are exacerbated by producers marketing strategies; for instance, SABMiller spent US$74.5 million on advertising alcohol in South Africa alone in 2010 (Jernigan & Babor, 2015). The marketing of alcohol by producers leads us to discuss the influence of alcohol producers.

Although most countries have implemented alcohol tax policies, they have not embraced WHO's alcohol control policies (i.e., the four regulatory categories; price, taxation, availability, marketing, and drink-driving measures) that are cost-effective (Morojele et al., 2021). Some countries implement insignificant alcohol controls (e.g., Zimbabwe) while others have total prohibitions (e.g., Libya, Somalia, Sudan, and Mauritania) (World

Health Organization, 2011). Majority of the countries have total bans against Muslim citizens only (e.g., Comoros, Maldives, and Mauritania).

The Influence of Alcohol Producers

The key producers in Africa include home-brewers who make and sell traditional brews, local industrial breweries, wineries and distillers, as well as global corporations who may operate under local industrial producers and/or import internationally produced alcoholic beverages (Jernigan & Babor, 2015). According to Jernigan & Babor et al. (2015), Africa's increasing population and urbanization make the continent attractive to global alcohol corporations. In fact, it is corporations such as SABMiller, AB InBev, and Diageo, that dominate alcohol production and supply and their size and profitability help to increase the demand, availability, and access to alcoholic beverages in Africa (Babor et al., 2015; Hanefeld et al., 2016; Jernigan & Babor, 2015). A case in point, these corporations have been complicit in preventing the formulation and implementation of comprehensive alcohol control policies and in promoting ineffective strategies (Ferreira-Borges et al., 2017). Bakke and Endal (2010) indicated that SABMiller and the International Center for Alcohol Policies assisted the governments of Lesotho, Malawi, Uganda, and Botswana to formulate their national alcohol control policies as a way to block any policy that might be a threat to their business interests. They did the same in South Africa with the proposal for a marketing ban on alcoholic beverages (Jernigan, 2013; Parry & Meyers, 2014) and with the 2016 Liquor Amendment Bill that intended to raise the drinking age.

Parry and Meyers (2014) suggested that governments need to make it clear that the alcohol industry has no role to play in the formulation of alcohol policies. Due to the clear conflicts of interest, partnerships with the alcohol industry should be avoided. Governments need to be sturdier in the design and implementation of policies and to resist pressures from alcohol corporations that continue to target sub-Saharan Africa. In addition, alcohol policies and restrictions should focus on evidence-based modalities and methods. Further research into the way alcohol policies are perceived should be a prerequisite so that the measures introduced have the envisioned effect (Sebeelo, 2020).

Global Strategy: Best Practices and Shortfalls on Policies that Help with Resisting Pressure from Alcohol Companies

The WHO ten key areas of policy alternatives and interventions that they considered as best practices for resisting pressures from alcohol corporations have been listed under the subheading National Alcohol Control Policies (WHO, 2019). Most of the listed key areas have been discussed in Chaps. 3, 4, and 7, focusing on best practices. Future papers could concentrate on leadership, awareness and commitment (1), community action (3), and monitoring and evaluation (10). Although most African countries have alcohol excise taxes, their governments have not adjusted for inflation, thereby gradually reducing the efficacy of these taxes, leading to consumer affordability (Peer, 2017). The aforementioned author also posited that most African countries do not have mandatory regulations for alcohol marketing, and those that have do not always implement them.

Nonetheless, the information on which African countries have implemented the strategies to control harmful alcohol consumption remains limited; thus, evaluations are needed to monitor progress towards implementing them and to identify areas where countries could strengthen their prevention policies (Ferreira-Borges et al., 2015). However, some authors have reviewed the alcohol policy environment in certain countries (e.g., South Africa) (Parry, 2010, 2014). Furthermore, Ferreira-Borges et al. (2017) proposed integrating alcohol education and treatment into primary health care, and ensuring that international trade treaties do not undermine efforts to control alcohol misuse by various countries.

Conclusion

Given the impact of alcohol misuse, governments and the international community have found it essential to control and prevent the harmful impact of alcohol through formulating policies and laws that curb its excessive use. Several evidence-based policy options have been discussed; for instance, regulating the alcohol availability (e.g., reducing outlet density, and decreasing days and hours of sales), reducing its affordability (e.g., increasing the price through taxation), putting restrictions on its marketing, and drinking and driving countermeasures (e.g., maximum limits on blood alcohol concentration [BAC]) (Babor, 2010). The policies are put forth after a thorough assessment of communities so that there is record of vulnerable communities that are usually a priority as they require urgent interventions (United Nations Office on Drugs and Crime, 2017). All policies must reach all citizens that need the intervention including youth in rural areas.

End of Chapter Questions

1. How can the effectiveness of alcohol policies be ascertained in sub-Saharan Africa?
2. What research areas could be explored looking at the environment of policies and the alcohol industries in sub-Saharan Africa?
3. Identify different alcohol policies in the different countries in Africa and discuss how the policies can be modified for efficacy.
4. How can we include young people in the formulation of efficacious alcohol policies?
5. How can governments be stern on alcohol producers to reduce alcohol marketing strategies bearing in mind the impact of alcohol on health and well-being?

References

African Development Bank – Department of Transport and ICT. (2013). *Road safety in Africa: Assessment of progress and challenges in road safety management system*. African Development Bank Group. https://www.afdb.org/fileadmin/uploads/afdb/Documents/Events/ATFforum/Road_Safety_in_Africa_-_Assesement_of_Progresses_and_Challenges_in_Road_Safety_-_AfDB.pdf

Arrive Alive. (n.d.). *Corruption, traffic enforcement and road safety*. https://www.arrivealive.mobi/corruption-traffic-enforcement-and-road-safety

Anderson, P., Chisholm, D., & Fuhr, D. C. (2009). Effectiveness and cost-effectiveness of policies and programmes to reduce the harm caused by alcohol. *Lancet, 373*(9682), 2234–2246. https://doi.org/10.1016/S0140-6736(09)60744-3

Babor, T. (2010). Public health science and the global strategy on alcohol. *Bulletin on World Health Organisation, 88*, 643.

Babor, T., Caetano, R., Casswell, S., et al. (2010). *Alcohol: No ordinary commodity. Research and public policy* (2nd ed.). Oxford University Press.

Babor, T., Robaina, K., & Jernigan, D. (2015). The influence of industry actions on the availability of alcoholic beverages in the African region. *Addiction, 110*, 561–571.

Bakke, O., & Endal, D. (2010). Vested interests in addiction research and policy alcohol policies out of context: Drinks industry supplanting government role in alcohol policies in sub-Saharan Africa. *Addiction, 105*, 22–28.

De Jong, M., Vonk, M., Jenkins, L. S., Reid, S., & Reuter, H. (2020). Prohibiting alcohol sales during the coronavirus disease 2019 pandemic has positive effects on health services in South Africa. *African Journal of Primary Health Care & Family Medicine, 12*(1), e1–e4. https://doi.org/10.4102/phcfm.v12i1.2528

Elder, R. W., Lawrence, B., Ferguson, A., Naimi, T. S., Brewer, R. D., Chattopadhyay, S. K., … Task Force on Community Preventive Services. (2010). The effectiveness of tax policy interventions for reducing excessive alcohol consumption and related harms. *American Journal of Preventive Medicine, 38*(2), 217–229.

Ferreira-Borges, C., Esser, M. B., Dias, S., Babor, T., & Parry, C. D. H. (2015). Alcohol control policies in 46 African countries: Opportunities for improvement. *Alcohol and Alcoholism, 50*(4), 470–476. https://doi.org/10.1093/alcalc/agv036

Ferreira-Borges, C., Ketsela, T., Munodawafa, D., & Alisalad, A. (2013). Reduction of the harmful use of alcohol: A strategy for the WHO African region. *African Health Monitor, 16*, 31–34.

Ferreira-Borges, C., Parry, C. D. H., & Babor, T. F. (2017). Harmful use of alcohol: A shadow over sub-Saharan Africa in need of workable solutions. *International Journal of Environmental Research and Public Health, 14*, 346. https://doi.org/10.3390/ijerph14040346

Hanefeld, J., Hawkins, B., Knai, C., Hofman, K., & Petticrew, M. (2016). What the InBev merger means for health in Africa. *BMJ Global Health, 1*. https://doi.org/10.1136/bmjgh-2016-000099

Jernigan, D. (2013). Why South Africa's proposed advertising ban matters. *Addiction, 108*, 1183–1185.

Jernigan, D., & Babor, T. (2015). The concentration of the global alcohol industry and its penetration in the African region. *Addiction, 110*, 551–560.

Kalema, D. (2019, October 20). *The long journey to alcohol policy in Uganda*. Movendi International. https://www.movendi.ngo/news/2019/09/26/uganda-cabinet-approves-alcohol-control-policy/

Masupe, T., Mochankana, K., Masole, U., & Kuate, L. (2017). *The impact of implementation of alcohol levy amongst drinkers in Gaborone, Botswana: Is it time for a national rehabilitation Centre?* University of Botswana. https://www.researchgate.net/publication/321475318_The_impact_of_implementation_of_alcohol_levy_amongst_drinkers_in_Gaborone_Botswana_Is_it_time_for_a_national_rehabilitation_Centre/link/5a22d2a1a6fdcc8e8666d30e/download

Matanje Mwagomba, B. L., Nkhata, M. J., Baldacchino, A., Wisdom, J., & Ngwira, B. (2018). Alcohol policies in Malawi: Inclusion of WHO "best buy" interventions and use of multi- sectoral action. *BMC Public Health, 18*(Supplementary 1), 957–968. https://doi.org/10.1186/s12889-018-5833-7

Middleton, J. C., Hahn, R. A., Kuzara, J. L., Elder, R., Brewer, R., Chattopadhyay, S., … Lawrence, B. (2010). Effectiveness of policies maintaining or restricting days of alcohol sales on excessive alcohol consumption and related harms. *American Journal of Preventive Medicine, 39*(6), 575–589.

Morojele, N. K., Dumbili, E. W., Obot, I. S., & Parry, C. D. H. (2021). Alcohol consumption, harms, and policy developments in sub-Saharan Africa: The case for stronger national and regional responses. *Drug Alcohol Review, 40*, 402–419. https://doi.org/10.1111/dar.13247

Moss, H. B. (2013). The impact of alcohol on society: A brief overview. *Social Work in Public Health, 28*(3-4), 175–177.

Muscat, R., & Pike, B. (2012). *Reflections on the concept of coherency for a policy on psychoactive substances and beyond.* Council of Europe Publishing.

Okwe, M. (2016), December 29. *Government raises import duties on consumable, luxury goods.* http://guardian.ng/news/government-raises-import-duties-on-consumable- luxury-goods/.

Olawole-Isaac, A., Ogundipe, O., Amoo, E. O., & Adeloye, D. (2018). Substance use among adolescents in sub-Saharan Africa: A systematic review and meta-analysis. South African Journal of Child Health, 12, s79–s84. https://doi.org/10.7196/sajch.2018.v12i2.1524

Parry, C. (2010). Alcohol policy in South Africa: A review of policy development processes between 1994 and 2009. *Addiction, 105*, 1340–1345.

Parry, C. (2014). Testing the National Alcohol Policy Score Card (NAPSC) to assess progress in implementing a comprehensive policy response to reduce the harmful use of alcohol in South Africa. *International Journal of Alcohol and Drug Research, 3*, 202–209.

Parry, C., Burnhams, N. H., & London, L. (2012). A total ban on alcohol advertising: Presenting the public health case. *South African Medical Journal, 102*(7), 602–604. https://doi.org/10.7196/SAMJ.5945

Parry, C., & Meyers, B. (2014). Delays in South Africa's plans to ban alcohol advertising. *Lancet, 383*, 1972–1972.

Peer, N. (2017). There has been little progress in implementing comprehensive alcohol control strategies in Africa. *The American Journal of Drug and Alcohol Abuse, 43*(6), 631–635. https://doi.org/10.1080/00952990.2017.1316986

Pitso, J. M. N., & Obot, I. S. (2011). Botswana alcohol policy and the presidential levy controversy. *Addiction, 106*, 898–905. https://doi.org/10.1111/j.1360-0443.2011.03365.x

Ramsoomar, L., & Morojele, N. K. (2012). Trends in alcohol prevalence, age of initiation and association with alcohol-related harm among south African youth: Implications for policy. *South African Medical Journal, 102*, 609–612.

Rehm, J., Taylor, B., & Room, R. (2006). Global burden of disease from alcohol, illicit drugs and tobacco. *Drug Alcohol Review, 25*, 503–513.

Saxena, S., Sharma, R. A. J., & Maulik, P. K. (2003). Impact of alcohol use on poor families: A study from North India. *Journal of Substance Use, 8*(2), 78–84.

Sebeelo, T. (2020). Beer drinking, resistance and the politics of the alcohol tax levy in Botswana. *Nordic Studies on Alcohol and Drugs, 37*(6), 544–556. https://doi.org/10.1177/1455072520936811

Sifile, L. (2016, May 17). *Nafcoc will fight proposed increase in minimum drinking age*. http://www.timeslive.co.za/local/2016/05/17/Nafcoc-will-fight-proposed-increase-in-minimum-drinking-age

South Africa Department of Trade & Industry. (2016). *Draft liquor amendment bill*. South African Government Gazette. https://www.gov.za/documents/liquor-amendment-bill-draft-30-sep-2016-0000

South Africa Department of Transport. (2015). *National road traffic amendment bill*. South African Government Gazette. https://www.gov.za/documents/national-road-traffic-amendment-bill-draft-28jan2015

Staton, C. A., Vissoci, J. R. N., Toomey, N., Abdelgadir, J., Chou, P., Haglund, M., … Swahn, M. (2018). The impact of alcohol among injury patients in Moshi, Tanzania: A nested case-crossover study. *BMC Public Health, 18*(1), 275. https://doi.org/10.1186/s12889-018-5144-z

Swahn, M.H., Ali, B., Palmier, J.B., Sikazwe, G., & Mayeya, J. (2011). Alcohol marketing, drunkenness, and problem drinking among Zambian youth: Findings from the 2004 Global School-Based Student Health Survey. *Journal of Environmental and Public* Health, 2011. https://doi.org/10.1155/2011/497827.

Thavorncharoensap, M., Teerawattananon, Y., Yothasamut, J., & Lertpitakpong, C. (2009). The economic impact of alcohol consumption: A systematic review. *Substance Abuse Treatment, Prevention, and Policy, 4*(1), 1–11.

U.S. Department of Health and Human Services. (2016). *The surgeon general's report on alcohol, drugs, and health*. U.S. Department of Health and Human Services.

United Nations Development Programme. (2017). *Desk review of the Botswana National Alcohol Policy: Final report*. UNDP Botswana Country Office. https://info.undp.org

United Nations Office on Drugs and Crime. (2017). World Drug Report. United Nations Publication, eISBN: 978-92-1-060623-3.

Vandenberg, B., Jiang, H., & Livingston, M. (2019). Effects of changes to the taxation of beer on alcohol consumption and government revenue in Australia. *International Journal of Drug Policy, 70*, 1–7.

Wagenaar, A. C., Salois, M. J., & Komro, K. A. (2009). Effects of beverage alcohol price and tax levels on drinking: A meta-analysis of 1003 estimates from 112 studies. *Addiction, 104*(2), 179–190.

Wagenaar, C. A., Tobler, A. L., & Komro, K. A. (2010). Effects of alcohol tax and price policies on morbidity and mortality: A systematic review. *American Journal of Public Health, 100*(2), 2270–2278.

World Health Organization. (2017, August). *Malawi launches the National Alcohol Policy.* https://www.afro.who.int/news/malawi-launches-national-alcohol-policy-18-august-2017

Willis, J. (2006). Drinking crisis? Change and continuity in cultures of drinking in sub-Saharan Africa. *African Journal of Drug & Alcohol Studies, 5*(1), 1–15.

World Health Organisation. (2009). *Evidence for the effectiveness and cost-effectiveness of interventions to reduce alcohol-related harm.* World Health Organisation.

World Health Organisation. (2010). *Global strategy to reduce the harmful use of alcohol.* World Health Organisation.

World Health Organisation Regional Office for Africa. (2010). *Reduction of the harmful use of alcohol: A strategy for the WHO African region.* World Health Organisation Regional Office for Africa.

World Health Organization. (2011). *Global status report on alcohol and health, 2011.* World Health Organization.

World Health Organization. (2014). *Global status report on alcohol and health, 2014.* World Health Organization.

World Health Organization. (2018). *Global status report on alcohol and health, 2018.* World Health Organization. https://apps.who.int/iris/handle/10665/274603

Xu, X., & Chaloupka, F. J. (2011). The effects of prices on alcohol use and its consequences. *Alcohol Research and Health, 34*(2), 236–245.

Xu, Y., Yu, Q., Scribner, R., Theall, K., Scribner, S., & Simonsen, N. (2012). Multilevel spatiotemporal change-point models for evaluating the effect of an alcohol outlet control policy on changes in neighborhood assaultive violence rates. *Spatial and Spatio-temporal Epidemiology, 3*(2), 121–128. https://doi.org/10.1016/j.sste.2012.04.005

Xuan, Z., Blanchette, J. G., Nelson, T. F., Nguyen, T. H., Hadland, S. E., Oussayef, N. L., ... Naimi, T. S. (2015). Youth drinking in the United States: Relationships with alcohol policies and adult drinking. *Pediatrics, 136*(1), 18–27.

Yu, Q., Scribner, R., Carlin, B., Theall, K., Simonsen, N., Ghosh-Dastidar, B., ... Mason, K. (2008). Multilevel spatio-temporal dual change point models for relating alcohol outlet destruction and changes in neighbourhood rates of assaultive violence. *Geospatial Health, 2*(2), 161–172.

CHAPTER 5

Tobacco: A Looming Epidemic in Sub-Saharan African Countries

Bontle Mbongwe and Roy Tapera

Abstract Sub-Saharan Africa, a region already burdened with HIV/AIDS, other infectious diseases, and competing priorities, is battling with the increasing burden of COVID-19 and non-communicable diseases (e.g., cardiovascular diseases, lung cancer). Africa's statistics on young people aged 13–15 years already hooked to tobacco are at an alarming 17%, matching the global trend. It is estimated that the number of smokers in sub-Saharan Africa will increase to 208 million (148%) by 2030, if robust tobacco control measures are not implemented. The chapter highlights the global trends of tobacco use, and exposure to tobacco smoke, all of which aggravate the prevalence of communicable and non-communicable diseases. The chapter also explores the harmful impact of tobacco use on people's health, suggesting that tobacco control should be a public health priority. The chapter presents the evidence for effective community-based interventions on tobacco control and prevention to reverse the tobacco epidemic in sub-Saharan Africa.

B. Mbongwe (✉) • R. Tapera
Department of Environmental Health, School of Public Health, University of Botswana, Gaborone, Botswana
e-mail: mbongwe@ub.ac.bw; taperar@ub.ac.bw

M. Mhaka-Mutepfa (ed.), *Substance Use and Misuse in sub-Saharan Africa*, https://doi.org/10.1007/978-3-030-85732-5_5

Keywords Tobacco use • Youth • Sustainable development goals • Non-communicable diseases • Covid-19 • HIV and AIDS • Environmental tobacco smoke • Impact on health

Global Trends of Tobacco Use

Over eight million premature fatalities have been recorded due to tobacco-related diseases worldwide (World Health Organization [WHO], 2019). These fatalities are projected to rise due to the long incubation period of tobacco-related conditions after exposure. While the estimated prevalence of tobacco smoking by regions has been going down slightly (see Fig. 5.1), the number of smokers continues to increase due to the global population growth (Navas-Acien, 2018) and several other factors. Of major concern is that there is no safe level of tobacco exposure. In 2015, a quarter of the global population were tobacco users (males 40.3% and females 9.5%). Assuming that current efforts in tobacco control are maintained in all countries, the rate is projected to decline further to a fifth (30%) of the

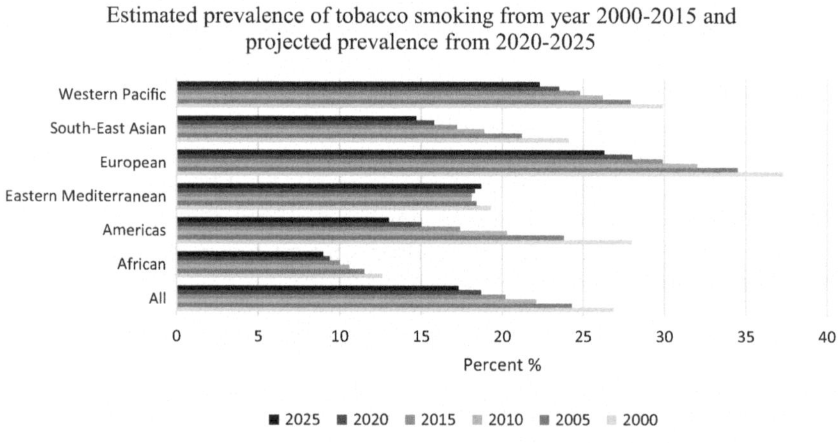

Fig. 5.1 Global trends in current tobacco use among people aged ≥15 years (WHO, 2019)

global population (males 35% and females 8%) by 2025 (WHO, 2019). The South-East Asian region had the highest prevalence of tobacco use (31.2%) in 2015 and is projected to have fallen to 25.1% in 2025. This is followed by countries in Europe (27.4%), where the prevalence was 13.5% in 2015, and is projected to decline to 11.2% by 2025. More needs to be done for reduction of users to continue and last.

Tobacco Use in Developing Countries

The prevalence of tobacco use is high among adults in some developing countries like Bangladesh (35.3%). At the same time, exposure to second-hand smoke in homes, restaurants, and public transportation is 39.0%, 49.7%, and 44.0%, respectively (Global Adult Tobacco Survey [GATS], 2017a). In India, 28.6% of all adults currently use tobacco (smoked and/or smokeless tobacco), while 38.7% of adults are exposed to second-hand smoke (GATS, 2017c). Nonetheless, the target for reducing tobacco use was pegged at 18.5% in Africa against a global target of 10.4% (WHO, 2014a), which needs perseverance to achieve. Tobacco use involves the use of all tobacco products which are associated with adverse health outcomes (Siddiqi, 2019). The impact of tobacco on health is discussed in detail in Chap. 7.

Tobacco products refer to merchandises entirely or partly made from the leaf tobacco as a raw material and may be used for smoking, sucking, chewing, or snuffing (WHO, 2014a). Out of the more than eight million people who die each year globally due to consumption of tobacco, seven million deaths occur because of direct tobacco use, whilst 1.2 million are a result of exposure to second-hand tobacco smoke (WHO, 2020). Second-hand smoke is smoke from burning tobacco products, such as cigarettes, cigars, or pipes and includes smoke that has been exhaled or breathed out by the smoking person (Suarez-Torres et al., 2020; United States Department of Health and Human Services [HHS], 2014).

Table 5.1 shows the top five countries with the highest prevalence of tobacco users in sub-Saharan Africa in terms of total tobacco use prevalence, the prevalence of smoking tobacco products including cigarettes, cigars and others, and the prevalence of smoking cigarettes only (see WHO, 2019).

Additional statistics indicate that, in Botswana, 13.8% of adults were exposed to tobacco smoke at home, 67.4% were exposed in bars and night

Table 5.1 Overall tobacco use, overall smoking, and cigarette smoking, adjusted prevalence (%) among people aged 15 years and older in sub-Saharan Africa

Tobacco use prevalence		*Smoking prevalence (any smoked tobacco product)*		*Cigarette smoking prevalence*	
South Africa	30.9	Lesotho	26.1	Lesotho	22.6
Lesotho	28.9	Seychelles	21.2	Mauritius	18.9
Madagascar	28.3	Mauritius	21.1	Seychelles	18.2
Mauritius	26.1	Madagascar	20.2	South Africa	16.6
Botswana	23.4	South Africa	20.3	Sierra Leone	15.1

WHO (2019)

clubs, 7.5% in public transportation, and 12.5% in enclosed areas at their workplaces (GATS, 2017b). In Kenya, the overall tobacco use is 11.6%, while 86.7% of adults who visited night clubs and bars were exposed to second-hand smoke, 17.7% of those who worked indoors were exposed to second-hand smoke, and 21.2% in restaurants (GATS, 2014). Ethiopia has a relatively low adult tobacco use prevalence of 5%, 3.7% smoke tobacco products, and 12.6% are exposed to second-hand smoke at home (GATS, 2016). Among adults who worked indoors in Ethiopia, 29.3% of them were exposed to tobacco smoke at the workplace (GATS, 2016).

Similar to Ethiopia, Nigeria has a low prevalence with 5.6% of its population using tobacco products, 3.9% smoking them, with 17.3% of indoor workers exposed to tobacco smoke, while 6.6% were exposed at home, and 29.3% at restaurants (GATS, 2012). Regarding the youth, 2.8% smoke cigarettes in Ghana, and 6.4% use tobacco products (GYTS, 2011). In contrast, 21.5% of students in South Africa were using some form of tobacco, 12.7% smoked cigarettes, 13.5% used some other form of tobacco, and 29% were exposed to second-hand smoke in their homes (GYTS, 2011). Lesotho had a slightly higher prevalence with 24.8% of youth using tobacco products, 10.1% smoking, and 36.9% exposed to second-hand smoke at home (GYTS, 2008). Despite the aforementioned high prevalence of tobacco use, there are other emerging tobacco products.

Emerging Tobacco Products

The use of several leading novel and emerging nicotine and tobacco products other than conventional cigarettes is on the increase (Navas-Acien, 2018). According to WHO (2014), these can be classified into electronic nicotine delivery systems (ENDS), electronic non-nicotine delivery systems (ENNDS) and heated tobacco products (HTPs). WHO recommends that the foregoing products must be regulated to mitigate penetration in national markets as they could threaten the implementation of the WHO Framework on Tobacco Control (WHO FCTC) (WHO, 2019). The WHO FCTC is discussed in detail in Chap. 6.

New tobacco products such as electronic cigarettes (e-cigarettes) are popular among young people, and waterpipe (hookah, narghile, or shisha) is common among Middle Eastern countries, the USA, and Western countries (Maziak et al., 2015). In a study done in 13 countries, Vietnam had the highest prevalence of waterpipe use (13.0%), followed by Egypt (6.2%) among those 15 years and above. In 2014, the use of water pipes among women was highest in Russia (3.2%) and Ukraine (1.1%) (Morton et al., 2014). These products are fuelled by tobacco companies and their marketing.

Case Study 5.1: Culture and Lifestyle, the Hidden Tobacco Advertising and Promotion Strategies

Shisha Lifestyle is a company that targets a collective of urban customers (21+ years) and aims to offer a more mature alternative service to the working, middle and upper class. Over the years, new terminology has been used for this form of smoking. The Americans call it *hookah*, the Persians call it *shisha* and South Africans call it *hubbly bubbly* (syrup tobacco mix containing molasses and vegetable glycerol smoke). Shisha Lifestyle is for those seeking pleasure and euphoria. The flavours contain flavoured molasses which mask the tobacco smell making the hubbly bubbly less irritating compared to the other tobacco products. However, it has side effects, a typical tobacco hookah session contains up to 200 puffs and one regular cigarette contains 20 puffs. The volume of smoke inhaled is up to 900,000 milliliters unlike the 500 millimeters of a cigarette. Shisha in some aspects may be seen as harmful, it however joins various Indian, Persian, Arabian customs, western contemporary culture and the developing Botswana culture.

Adapted from Online Editor (2016).

Stop and Reflect

1. Discuss the current tobacco use status in sub-Saharan Africa.
2. What are the emerging and re-emerging tobacco products, and who are the targets?
3. Why do marketers use names like hubbly bubbly when advertising shisha?
4. What is your view of above case study?

The Burden of Disease Due to Tobacco Use

Evidence shows that tobacco smoke contains more than 7000 chemicals, and several toxins, 70 of which cause cancer (United States Department of Health and Human Services, 2014). The burden of tobacco consumption on non-communicable diseases (NCDs), on people living with HIV, and communicable diseases such as tuberculosis (TB) and coronavirus are discussed.

Non-Communicable Diseases (NCDs) and Tobacco Use

NCDs are the leading cause of death globally. According to the WHO (2018), 41 million of the world's 57 million deaths were attributable to NCDs in 2016 and 15 million of the deaths affected adults aged 30–70 years (classified as premature deaths). Unlike in the past, where communicable diseases were the leading cause of morbidity and mortality in low-income countries, NCDs, fuelled by the consumption of tobacco and other lifestyle issues, are projected to surpass communicable diseases by 2030 (World Health Organization, 2014b). Cardiovascular diseases (CVDs), type 2 diabetes mellitus (T2DM), chronic respiratory diseases, and cancer contributed to nearly 80% of all NCD deaths worldwide in 2016 (WHO, 2018). There is also evidence that smoking significantly increases the risk of diabetic foot amputation compared with non-smoking (Liu et al., 2018).

Case Study 5.2: The Impact of Smoking on Amputations
A consultant surgeon has raised concern over tobacco smoking, saying it is the cause of most amputations performed at a hospital in Botswana. He claimed that 13 out of 14 patients had their limbs amputated as a result of smoking the previous year. He reiterated that smoking is a deadly habit, which should be discouraged at all costs because smoking constricts blood movement leading to the death of tissues in a limb leading to amputation. The surgeon feels there is still a strong need for more campaigns to sensitise the public on the hazards of smoking. He pleaded with tobacco smokers to quit the habit as it is hazardous to their lives hence a change in lifestyle is essential. He applauded the Botswana government for banning smoking in public areas, adding that such a decision is a step in the right direction. The surgeon also warned people who are HIV positive to desist from smoking as they have a higher chance of getting their limbs amputated.

Adapted from Online Editor (2013).

Stop and Reflect

1. What other health complications does tobacco use cause? Discuss.
2. Discuss whether smokers abide by restrictions of smoking in public places in your communities. How can the restrictions be enforced?
3. Why are people who smoke prone to amputations than those who do not smoke?
4. Discuss the negative impact of tobacco on other diseases or conditions in your community.

The WHO (2019) estimates that 1.3 billion people use tobacco globally, and 80% of these live in low- and middle-income countries (LMICs). Of particular concern is that tobacco consumption is the single most preventable cause of cardiovascular diseases (CVDs) and other chronic illnesses, including the overall population health. It is still widely used by both the young and old globally (WHO, 2019). Tobacco use is a common risk factor to the main NCDs such as CVDs, cancer, chronic respiratory disease, including neurological disorders (WHO, 2018). The use of tobacco, including smoking and using smokeless tobacco, is the leading risk factor for illness and death from major NCDs (WHO, 2020). Increasing rates of smoking in many LMICs and decreasing rates in high-income countries (HICs) may lead to increased proportional tobacco-related mortality in LMICs. LMICs were leading, recording 78% of all NCD deaths (WHO, 2018).

The harm caused by tobacco results from direct consumption of smoking and nonsmokers' exposure to second-hand smoke or environmental tobacco smoke (Suarez-Torres et al., 2020). Smokeless tobacco is carcinogenic to its users; with the oral cavity incurring the most harm as it is where the products are applied locally (Cai et al., 2020).

Communicable Diseases and Tobacco Use

Tobacco use complicates other diseases. This section focuses on communicable diseases; TB, HIV/AIDS, and Covid-19.

Tobacco Consumption and Effects on TB Treatment There is substantial evidence that tobacco smoking is associated with an increased risk of TB infection and TB disease (Lin et al., 2007; WHO, 2009a). Evidence also shows a relationship between adverse effects of tobacco consumption on TB related deaths (Lin et al., 2007; WHO, 2009b) and TB outcomes in patients with established TB. Tobacco smoking not only affects the disease outcomes but is also associated with relapse and death during or after treatment, lower treatment adherence, and TB treatment failure, among other factors (Chiang et al., 2012; Maciel et al., 2013). Of major concern is the joint effects of smoking, TB, and HIV, which aggravate the risk of chronic obstructive pulmonary disease (COPD) over time (van Zyl Smit et al., 2010).

Tobacco Consumption, the Immune System, and HIV/AIDS Tobacco and tobacco smoke compromises the equilibrium, or balance, of the immune system. This characteristic increases the risk for several adverse conditions, including lung cancer, caused when the immune system mistakenly attacks the body's healthy cells and tissues or autoimmune disorders (Yamaguchi, 2019). Further evidence shows that smoking is a cause of rheumatoid arthritis, an autoimmune disease in which the immune system attacks the joints and causes swelling and pain (Chang et al., 2014).

Smoking and people living with HIV/AIDS (PLWHA) may lead to a challenged immune system as both target the immune system (Yamaguchi, 2019). Compared to people who never smoked, smokers, in general, suffer more health problems and die a decade or earlier than nonsmokers (WHO, 2018). Even without HIV/AIDS, smoking harms everyone's immune system, making the body less successful in fighting diseases (WHO, 2018). Tobacco and tobacco smoke may also have adverse effects on the immune response to anti-retroviral treatment (ART). Evidence shows that, compared to nonsmokers, smokers on ART have a reduced chance of achieving suppression of HIV viral load and therefore suffer immunological failure because CD4 cell count falls below pre-ART nadir levels (Pool et al., 2014).

The 7000 chemical compounds found in tobacco smoke contribute to significant morbidity and mortality among PLWHA. Evidence from studies of PLWHA revealed that smoking is attributable to 24.3% of all-cause mortality, 25.3% of major CVD, 30.6% of non-AIDS-related cancer, and 25.4% of bacterial pneumonia (Lifson et al., 2010). In addition, among PLWHA, lung cancer is the commonest non-AIDS-related cancer (Smith et al., 2018), and lung cancer occurs at a younger age, following a shorter period of exposure to tobacco, particularly cigarettes (Winston et al., 2013). Tobacco smoking aggravates CVD risk and acute coronary syndrome among PLWHA (Calvo-Sánchez et al., 2013; Petoumenos et al., 2011).

Quitting smoking has been identified as an effective intervention in reversing the risk among PLWHA (Petoumenos et al., 2011). Unlike in nonsmoking PLWHA, smoking increases the incidence of oral lesions such as oral candidiasis and oral hairy leukoplakia (de Souza et al., 2018), and the risk of bacterial pneumonia (Bénard et al., 2010). Also, it exacerbates the outcome of COPD (Morris et al., 2011). There is also compelling evidence that compared to general smokers, PLWHA and smoke are highly addicted to nicotine and, therefore, have a higher prevalence of other addictive substances such as alcohol and illicit drugs (Bénard et al., 2010). Therefore, they would be more vulnerable to cessation withdrawal symptoms and have difficulties sustaining abstinence, unlike their counterparts.

Smoking and Severity of COVID-19 COVID-19 is primarily a disease affecting the respiratory system and smokers are more vulnerable to developing severe COVID-19, resulting in death or prolonged hospitalisation on life support machines (Li et al., 2020). There is compelling evidence from previous studies that smokers are twice as likely to contract influenza and have more severe symptoms compared to nonsmokers (Han et al., 2019). While smokers were also noted to have higher mortality in the previous Middle East respiratory syndrome-related coronavirus (MERS-CoV) outbreak, emerging data from patients hospitalised with severe COVID-19 show higher percentages of current and former smokers among patients that have needed oxygen support, mechanical ventilation, or have died (Reddy et al., 2021). Thus, a higher percentage of smokers are among the severe cases. The impact of tobacco on health calls for effective intervention to curb the scourge.

Effective Community-Based Interventions for Tobacco Control

Community-based interventions on tobacco control are crucial to discourage tobacco use among individuals, families, and the community in developing nations (Hill et al., 2014). Interventions may include organising community groups to advocate the adoption of tobacco control regulations or policies such as enforcement bans on tobacco advertising, promotion, and sponsorship (see Case Study 5.3), point of sale advertising, smoking in public places such as restaurants and bars, the sale of tobacco products to minors, and others (Wilson et al., 2012).

Some of the key interventions strongly supported by governments include laws and policies protecting people from tobacco smoke (Drope et al., 2018). There is evidence that smoke-free policies reduce smoking behaviour, second-hand smoke exposure, and adverse health outcomes (Drope et al., 2018). While smoke-free laws and regulations are recognised as key in protecting public health, current research shows that more than 80% of the world's population is not protected by such policies (Drope et al., 2018). As a result, the WHO recommends that all countries adopt comprehensive smoke-free policies with no exemptions for venue types or allowances for designated smoking areas (WHO, 2004). Countries, particularly developed nations, have adopted policies and regulations on tobacco products packaging with large pictorial health warnings. Health warning labels have decreased smoking behaviour, resulting in reductions in tobacco use and increased motivation to quit among tobacco users (Hammond, 2011).

Case Study 5.3: Marketing of Tobacco Products to Minors

In an effort to increase access to tobacco products, the tobacco industry has developed attractive tobacco packaging for the sale of single cigarettes in some countries. In Botswana, custom made convenience packages that have a lighter are sold near schools to promote smoking (Mbongwe et al., 2018) (see *Free Cigarette Box (with lighters)*.

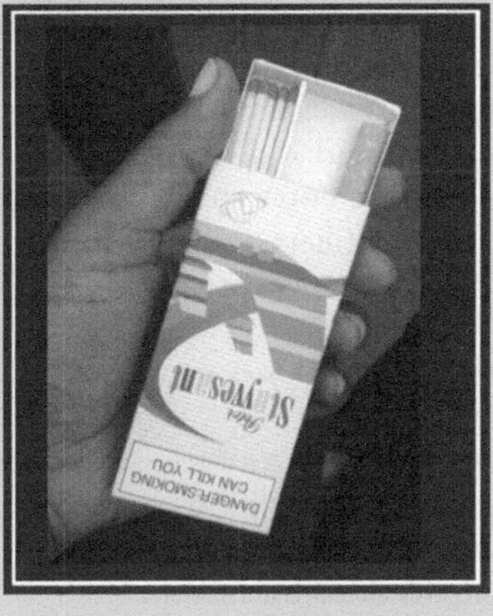

Stop and Reflect

1. Do fear-inducing pictorial presentations help in discouraging people from smoking? Discuss.
2. What other methods would you use to discourage your peers from using tobacco products?
3. How can the government intervene in eradicating scenes described in the case study above?

Conclusion

Other than the cigarette, which is the most common form of tobacco known for the harms it causes to human health, there are other equally harmful tobacco products such as waterpipe tobacco (shisha), smokeless tobacco, cigars, cigarillos, roll-your-own tobacco, pipe tobacco, and many others. Even though there are different ways to smoke cigarettes or consume tobacco, such as the "bidi" in India, and varying risk levels for each, smokers are still more vulnerable to the various health risks as compared to nonsmokers (Magitta, 2018). Contrary to popular beliefs among smokers, there is no 'safe level' of smoking, and the only way for one to avoid the health risks is to completely stop smoking.

Furthermore, while there is indisputable evidence that tobacco use causes heart disease, cancer, respiratory, and other NCDs, the early signs of these diseases are hardly detected. Tobacco use, therefore, affects both the young and old, smokers and nonsmokers. As a result, stakeholders should make concerted effort to prevent and intervene early to curb its deleterious effects. Prevention and intervention of substance use and other harmful substances are discussed in detail in Chaps. 12 and 13.

End of Chapter Questions

1. Discuss how countries can reduce tobacco consumption among the youth in developing countries.
2. Discuss any cultural uses of tobacco that you are aware of and their implications for health.
3. Why is tobacco smoking and exposure to tobacco smoke significant in the severity of Covid-19 and other diseases?
4. In your own experience, how has the tobacco industry targeted the youth in promoting tobacco use?
5. Smoke contains carbon monoxide and other chemicals which increase health risk. What other impact does smoking have on health? Discuss.

References

Bénard, A., Mercié, P., Alioum, A., Bonnet, F., Lazaro, E., Dupon, M., Neau, D., Dabis, F., Chêne, G., Dabis, F., Dupon, M., Longy-Boursier, M., Morlat, P., Pellegrin, J. L., Ragnaud, J. M., Bruyand, M., Chêne, G., Dabis, F., Lawson-Ayayi, S., ... Touchard, D. (2010). Bacterial pneumonia among HIV-infected patients: Decreased risk after tobacco smoking cessation. ANRS CO3 aquitaine cohort, 2000-2007. *PLoS One*, *5*(1). https://doi.org/10.1371/journal.pone.0008896

Cai, H., Xu, Y., Tang, S., Yang, X., Zou, Y., Wang, X., Mo, L., Wu, B., Liang, Z., Li, Y., Wei, X., Ao, Q., Meng, L., Zhang, N., Chen, M., Lan, C., Li, X., & Lu, C. (2020). Systemic toxicity evaluation of novel tobacco products in Caenorhabditis elegans. *Toxicology In Vitro, 62.* https://doi.org/10.1016/j.tiv.2019.104671.

Calvo-Sánchez, M., Perelló, R., Pérez, I., Mateo, M. G., Junyent, M., Laguno, M., Blanco, J. L., Martínez-Rebollar, M., Sánchez, M., Mallolas, J., Gatell, J. M., Domingo, P., & Martínez, E. (2013). Differences between HIV-infected and uninfected adults in the contributions of smoking, diabetes and hypertension to acute coronary syndrome: Two parallel case-control studies. *HIV Medicine,14*(1),40–48.https://doi.org/10.1111/j.1468-1293.2012.01057.x

Chang, K., Yang, S. M., Kim, S. H., Han, K. H., Park, S. J., & Shin, J. I. (2014). Smoking and rheumatoid arthritis. *International Journal of Molecular Sciences, 15*(12), 22279–22295. https://doi.org/10.3390/ijms151222279.

Chiang, Y. C., Lin, Y. M., Lee, J. A., Lee, C. N., & Chen, H. Y. (2012). Tobacco consumption is a reversible risk factor associated with reduced successful treatment outcomes of anti-tuberculosis therapy. *International Journal of Infectious Diseases, 16*(2) https://doi.org/10.1016/j.ijid.2011.10.007.

de Souza, A. J., Gomes-Filho, I. S., da Silva, C. A. L., de Santana Passos-Soares, J., da Cruz, S. S., Trindade, S. C., Figueiredo, A. C. M. G., de Paiva Buischi, Y., Seymour, G. J., & de Moraes Marcillo Cerqueira, E. (2018). Factors associated with dental caries, periodontitis and intra-oral lesions in individuals with HIV/AIDS. *AIDS Care – Psychological and Socio-Medical Aspects of AIDS/HIV, 30*(5), 578–585. https://doi.org/10.1080/09540121.2017.1400640.

Drope, J., Schluger, N., Cahn, Z., Drope, J., Hamill, S., Islami, F., Liber, A., Nargis, N., & Stoklosa, M. (2018). *The tobacco atlas* (6th ed.). The American Cancer Society, and Vital Strategies. www.tobaccoatlas.org

GATS. (2012). *Global adult tobacco survey: Country report 2012 Nigeria*. Global Adult Tobacco Survey.

GATS. (2014). *Global adult tobacco survey factsheet: Kenya 2014*. Global Adult Tobacco Survey. http://global.tobaccofreekids.org/files/pdfs/en/GATS_Kenya_Fact_Sheet_2014.pdf

GATS. (2016). *Global adult tobacco survey factsheet Ethiopia 2016*. Global Adult Tobacco Survey.

GATS. (2017a). *Global adult tobacco survey: Comparison factsheet Bangladesh 2009 and 2017*. Global Adult Tobacco Survey.

GATS. (2017b). *Global adult tobacco survey Botswana 2017*. Global Adult Tobacco Survey.

GATS. (2017c). *Global adult tobacco survey factsheet: India 2016–17*. Global Adult Tobacco Survey. https://www.who.int/tobacco/surveillance/survey/gats/GATS_India_2016-17_FactSheet.pdf

GYTS. (2008). *Global youth tobacco survey Lesotho factsheet*. Global Youth Tobacco Survey. https://extranet.who.int/ncdsmicrodata/index.php/catalog/143

GYTS. (2011). *Global youth tobacco survey (13–15) South Africa factsheet*. Global Youth Tobacco Survey. https://www.tobaccofreekids.org/assets/global/pdfs/en/South_Africa_GYTS_en.pdf

Hammond, D. (2011). Health warning messages on tobacco products: A review. *Tobacco Control, 20*(5), 327–337. https://doi.org/10.1136/tc.2010.037630.

Han, L., Ran, J., Mak, Y. W., Suen, L. K. P., Lee, P. H., Peiris, J. S. M., & Yang, L. (2019). Smoking and influenza-associated morbidity and mortality: A systematic review and meta-analysis. *Epidemiology, 30*(3), 405–417. https://doi.org/10.1097/EDE.0000000000000984.

Hill, S., Amos, A., Clifford, D., & Platt, S. (2014). Impact of tobacco control interventions on socioeconomic inequalities in smoking: Review of the evidence. *Tobacco Control, 23*(e2), e89–e97. https://doi.org/10.1136/tobaccocontrol-2013-051110.

Li, J., Long, X., Zhang, Q., Fang, X., Li, N., Fedorova, B., Hu, S., Li, J., Xiong, N., & Lin, Z. (2020). Tobacco smoking confers risk for severe COVID-19 unexplainable by pulmonary imaging. *Journal of Internal Medicine*. https://doi.org/10.1111/joim.13190

Lifson, A. R., Neuhaus, J., Arribas, J. R., Van, B.-W., Den, M., Labriola, A. M., & Read, T. R. H. (2010). Smoking-related health risks among persons with HIV in the strategies for management of antiretroviral therapy clinical trial. *American Journal of Public Health, 100*(10), 1896–1903. https://doi.org/10.2105/AJPH.2009.188664.

Lin, H. H., Ezzati, M., & Murray, M. (2007). Tobacco smoke, indoor air pollution and tuberculosis: A systematic review and meta-analysis. *PLoS Medicine, 4*(1), 0173–0189. https://doi.org/10.1371/journal.pmed.0040020.

Liu, M., Zhang, W., Yan, Z., & Yuan, X. (2018). Smoking increases the risk of diabetic foot amputation: A meta-analysis. *Experimental and Therapeutic Medicine, 15*(2), 1680–1685.

Maciel, E. L. N., Brioschi, A. P., Peres, R. L., Guidoni, L. M., Ribeiro, F. K., Hadad, D. J., Vinhas, S. A., Zandonade, E., Palaci, M., Dietze, R., & Johnson, J. L. (2013). Smoking and 2-month culture conversion during anti-tuberculosis treatment. *International Journal of Tuberculosis and Lung Disease, 17*(2), 225–228. https://doi.org/10.5588/ijtld.12.0426.

Magitta, N. F. (2018). Epidemiology of tobacco use and dependence in sub-Saharan Africa: A systematic review. *Journal of Pulmonology and Clinical Research, 2(1)*, 9–15

Maziak, W., Taleb, Z. B., Bahelah, R., Islam, F., Jaber, R., Auf, R., & Salloum, R. G. (2015). The global epidemiology of waterpipe smoking. *Tobacco Control, 24*, i3–i12. https://doi.org/10.1136/tobaccocontrol-2014-051903.

Mbongwe, B., Tapera, R., Katlholo, T., Erick, P., Rahube, T., Nsebula, N., Mokgethi, I., Chuma, M., Boitumelo, K., Molebatsi, M., & Tumoyagae, T. (2018). *Situational analysis on tobacco control in Botswana*. University of Botswana.

Morris, A., George, M. P., Crothers, K., Huang, L., Lucht, L., Kessinger, C., & Kleerup, E. C. (2011). HIV and chronic obstructive pulmonary disease: Is it worse and why? *Proceedings of the American Thoracic Society, 8*(3), 320–325. https://doi.org/10.1513/pats.201006-045WR.

Morton, J., Song, Y., Fouad, H., El Awa, F., El Naga, R.A., Zhao, L., Palipudi, K., & Asma, S. (2014). Cross-country comparison of waterpipe use: Nationally representative data from 13 low and middle-income countries from the Global Adult Tobacco Survey (GATS).

Navas-Acien, A. (2018). Global tobacco use: Old and new products. *Annals of the American Thoracic Society, 15*(4), S69–S75. https://doi.org/10.1513/AnnalsATS.201711-874MG.

Online Editor. (2013, April 14). *Most amputations at Nyangabwe blamed on smoking.* https://www.sundaystandard.info/most-amputations-at-nyangabwe-hospital-blamed-on-smoking/

Online Editor. (2016, July 2014). *Shisha LifeStyle is the new way to smoke.* https://www.sundaystandard.info/shisha-lifestyle-is-the-new-way-to-smoke/

Petoumenos, K., Worm, S., Reiss, P., de Wit, S., d'Arminio Monforte, A., Sabin, C., Friis-Møller, N., Weber, R., Mercie, P., Pradier, C., El-Sadr, W., Kirk, O., Lundgren, J., & Law, M. (2011). Rates of cardiovascular disease following smoking cessation in patients with HIV infection: Results from the D:A:D study. *HIV Medicine, 12*(7), 412–421. https://doi.org/10.1111/j.1468-1293.2010.00901.x.

Pool, E. R. M., Dogar, O., & Siddiqi, K. (2014). Interventions for tobacco use cessation in people living with HIV and AIDS. *Cochrane Database of Systematic Reviews.* https://doi.org/10.1002/14651858.CD011120

Reddy, R. K., Charles, W. N., Sklavounos, A., Dutt, A., Seed, P. T., & Khajuria, A. (2021). The effect of smoking on COVID-19 severity: A systematic review and meta-analysis. *Journal of Medical Virology, 93*(2), 1045–1056. https://doi.org/10.1002/jmv.26389.

Siddiqi, K. (2019). Tobacco use in sub-Saharan Africa: The risks and challenges. *Nicotine and Tobacco Research, 21*(8), 999–1000. https://doi.org/10.1093/ntr/ntz086.

Smith, D. M., Salters, K. A., Eyawo, O., Franco-Villalobos, C., Jabbari, S., Wiseman, S. M., Press, N., Montaner, J. S. G., Man, S. F. P., Hull, M., & Hogg, R. S. (2018). Mortality among people living with HIV/AIDS with non-small-cell lung cancer in the modern HAART Era. *AIDS Care – Psychological and Socio-Medical Aspects of AIDS/HIV, 30*(7), 936–942. https://doi.org/10.1080/09540121.2018.1434120.

Suarez-Torres, J. D., Alzate, J. P., & Orjuela-Ramirez, M. E. (2020). The NTP Report on carcinogens: A valuable resource for public health, a challenge for regulatory science. *Journal of Applied Toxicology, 40*(1), 169–175. https://doi.org/10.1002/jat.3894.

United States Department of Health and Human Services. (2014). *The health consequences of smoking-50 years of progress: A report of the Surgeon General.* United States Department of Health and Human Services.

van Zyl Smit, R. N., Pai, M., Yew, W. W., Leung, C. C., Zumla, A., Bateman, E. D., & Dheda, K. (2010). Global lung health: The colliding epidemics of tuberculosis, tobacco smoking, HIV and COPD. *European Respiratory Journal, 35*(1), 27–33. https://doi.org/10.1183/09031936.00072909.

Wilson, L. M., Tang, E. A., Chander, G., Hutton, H. E., Odelola, O. A., Elf, J. L., Heckman-Stoddard, B. M., Bass, E. B., Little, E. A., Haberl, E. B., & Apelberg, B. J. (2012). Impact of tobacco control interventions on smoking initiation, cessation, and prevalence: A systematic review. *Journal of Environmental and Public Health, 2012*. https://doi.org/10.1155/2012/961724.

Winston, T. A., Man, S. F. P., Hull, M., Montaner, J. S., & Sin, D. D. (2013). Epidemic of lung cancer in patients with HIV infection. *Chest, 143*(2), 305–314. https://doi.org/10.1378/chest.12-1699.

World Health Organisation. (2004). *WHO framework convention on tobacco control*. WHO Regional Office for South-East Asia. https://apps.who.int/iris/bitstream/handle/10665/206081/B3677.pdf

World Health Organisation. (2009a). *Global status report on road safety: Time for action*. WHO Library Cataloguing-in-Publication Data (Vol. 13, Issue 5). http://ra.ocls.ca/ra/login.aspx?url=http://search.ebscohost.com/login.aspx?direct=true&db=enr&AN=56097888&site=ehost-live

World Health Organisation. (2009b). *Tuberculosis & tobacco*. World Health Organisation.

World Health Organisation. (2014a). Electronic nicotine delivery systems report. *World Health Organisation*. https://doi.org/10.1161/CIRCULATIONAHA.114.008545.7

World Health Organisation. (2014b). *Global Status Report on non-communicable diseases 2014*. World Health Organisation.

World Health Organisation. (2018). Non-communicable diseases country profiles 2018. *World Health Organisation. WHO*. https://doi.org/10.1002/9781119097136.part5

World Health Organisation. (2019). *WHO global report on trends in prevalence of tobacco use 2000–2025*. World Health Organisation. https://www.who.int/publications/i/item/who-global-report-on-trends-in-prevalence-of-tobacco-use-2000-2025-third-edition

World Health Organisation. (2020). *Tobacco*. World Health Organisation. https://www.who.int/news-room/fact-sheets/detail/tobacco

Yamaguchi, N. H. (2019). Smoking, immunity, and DNA damage. *Translational Lung Cancer Research, 8*, S3–S6. https://doi.org/10.21037/tlcr.2019.03.02

CHAPTER 6

The Tobacco Industry's Interference: A Vector of the Tobacco Epidemic

Roy Tapera, Thabo Katlholo, Leonne Mfolwe, and Bontle Mbongwe

Abstract The tobacco pandemic, spearheaded by the tobacco industry's targeted deceptive advertising, has over the years shifted away from established economies to low- and middle-income countries (LMICs). Scientific evidence has established that tobacco companies' advertising and promotion influence people, particularly children and the youth, to start using tobacco. Young people exposed to tobacco advertising and promotion find tobacco products more appealing, and therefore, their desire to use tobacco products is equally increased. The first section of this chapter

R. Tapera (✉) • B. Mbongwe
Department of Environmental Health, School of Public Health, University of Botswana, Gaborone, Botswana
e-mail: taperar@ub.ac.bw; mbongwe@ub.ac.bw

T. Katlholo
Anti Tobacco Network, University of Botswana, Gaborone, Botswana

L. Mfolwe
Department of Psychology, Faculty of Social Sciences, University of Botswana, Gaborone, Botswana
e-mail: mfolwel@ub.ac.bw

M. Mhaka-Mutepfa (ed.), *Substance Use and Misuse in sub-Saharan Africa*, https://doi.org/10.1007/978-3-030-85732-5_6

summarises the marketing strategies of tobacco companies in high-income countries from the 1930s and how the tobacco industry used medical doctors to endorse tobacco smoking. Evidence on the tobacco industry's trail of strategies to shift tobacco use from developed to developing countries is explored. The second section focuses on the global response to the tactics of the tobacco industry to interfere with public health policies. The WHO Framework Convention on Tobacco Control (WHO/FCTC) Articles 5.3 and 13 guidelines developed for countries to counter tobacco industry interference, advertising, and promotion are also discussed. MPOWER, a set of six cost-effective and high impact measures that help countries reduce demand for tobacco products is briefly discussed.

Keywords Tobacco Advertising and Promotion • Youth Smoking • Developing Countries • Academic performance • MPOWER • Cigarette candies • Tobacco industry interference

Introduction

The tobacco industry, as defined by the World Health Organization (World Health Organization, 2012, p. 6), "includes manufacturers, importers and distributors of tobacco products and processors of tobacco leaf". The main goal of the tobacco industry is to make profits directly or indirectly from their tobacco products. In maximising such profits, the tobacco industry products have resulted in a global epidemic, particularly in low- and middle-income countries (LMICs), increasing disability, morbidity, and mortality (Britton, 2017). Despite this knowledge, tobacco companies have sold tobacco products for decades and disputed the health costs of tobacco products to maintain profits (WHO, 2012). For a similar reason, the industry has spent billions of dollars on advertising and promoting tobacco products. Cigarettes, in particular, have been heavily advertised in high-income countries since the early 1930s. In countries such as the United States of America (USA), billions of dollars have been spent on advertising these products. The US Federal Trade Commission (FTC) reported that spending on the promotion of cigarettes between 1975 and 1983 increased from $490 million to $1.9 billion (Federal Trade Commission, 1986) and continued to increase, standing at $7.6 billion as of 2019 (Federal Trade Commission, 2021). These monies have been spent on various marketing strategies over the years.

The WHO/FCTC prescribes the total elimination of advertising and promotion of tobacco products, including all forms of sponsorship by tobacco companies (WHO, 2013). According to the science backed convention, the banishment of advertising and promotion of tobacco products would decrease consumption, thereby reducing tobacco-induced disease and loss of human lives (WHO, 2013).

Tobacco companies have countered these issues by the WHO/FCTC, arguing that consumption of tobacco products would not be increased by advertising and promotions (Goldberg et al., 2006). These authors indicated that the tobacco industry is adamant that advertising tobacco has a relatively weak "share of voice" in the advertising and promotion environment and therefore would not influence smoking behaviour among the youth. The aforementioned arguments which dispute the impact of tobacco advertising on youth smoking behaviour, are intended to portray tobacco companies as responsible entities (Goldberg et al., 2006).

Marketing Strategies of the Tobacco Industry

From the 1930s to the 1950s, the tobacco industry in the USA had marketing strategies that included the endorsement by physicians to assert that cigarettes were safe for health (Gardner & Brandt, 2006). When these assertions became a subject of contention, marketing was then shifted to cultural icons like the "Marlboro Man" in the mid-1950s, which attracted male users by associating the smoking of cigarettes with masculinity and independence (White et al., 2012). By the 1990s, the tobacco industry had also aggressively marketed smokeless tobacco through sporting activities (Ling et al., 2010). In recent years, tobacco companies such as British American Tobacco and Phillip Morris International have adapted similar strategies to promote new non-cigarette products through renewed sponsorship of sports races and campaigns such as "its time to unsmoke" on social media (Action on Smoking and Health, 2019; Vice, 2012).

The tobacco industry has also targeted children, youth and women in its marketing strategies. New products such as candy-like flavoured electronic cigarettes (e-cigarettes) have been developed to increase the appeal of tobacco smoking in children (Klein & St Clair, 2000; Vasiljevic et al., 2016). Further, research shows that during preconception and pregnancy, women preferred fruit and mint flavoured e-cigarettes (Stroud et al., 2019). Some studies have shown a general impression by different community groups that e-cigarettes and hookahs are healthier alternatives to traditional cigarette smoking (Kahr et al., 2015; Rahman et al., 2014).

The tobacco industry has been accused of quashing adverse findings from research and impeding successful efforts to avoid legislation and/or regulations supported by the confectionery trade (Klein & St Clair, 2000). While deceptive products such as cigarette candies are banned in high-income countries, they are still available in LMICs such as Botswana to entice children (see Fig. 6.1 below).

Additionally, the tobacco industry in sub-Saharan Africa has sponsored music festivals and other events to appeal to the youth (Patel et al., 2009). Other vendors are taking advantage of tobacco industry marketing and promotion by advertising tobacco products (e.g., in Zambia, Botswana, Nigeria, and South Africa) while at the same time advertising other events to their benefit (Mbongwe et al., 2018). They use other means like social media (e.g., Facebook) to lure young adults into participating in events and getting free shisha/hubbly bubbly sessions, as shown in Fig. 6.2 below. Some studies have shown that young people such as college students perceive non-conventional tobacco products such as e-cigarettes or shisha/hookah as less harmful than traditional cigarettes (Martinasek et al., 2019; Noland et al., 2016). On the other hand, there is evidence that people who smoke these products are at increased risk of developing diseases (e.g., pulmonary diseases, oesophagus and gastric cancers) as they

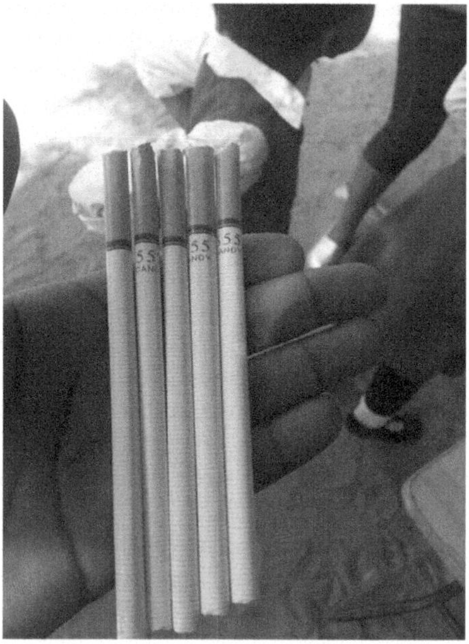

Fig. 6.1 Cigarette candies sold to children near primary schools (Mbongwe, 2019)

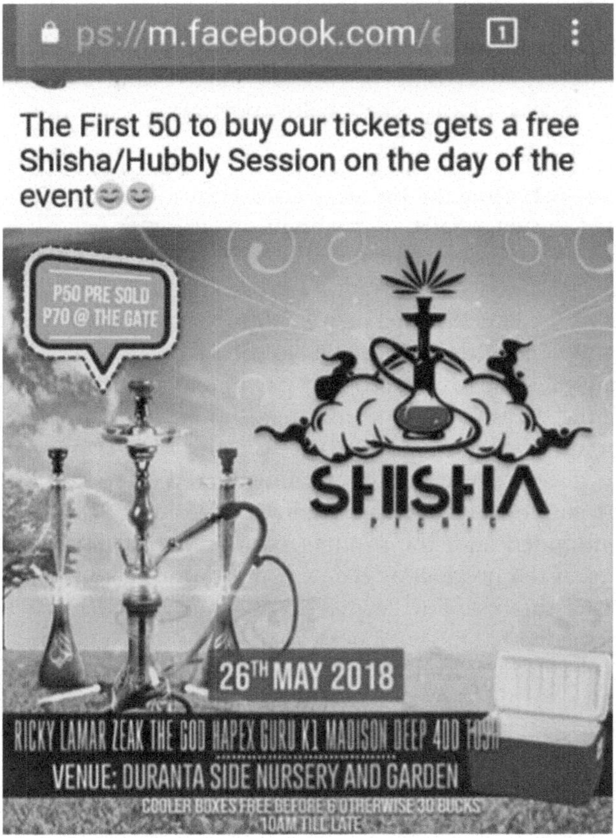

Fig. 6.2 Picture of Shisha advert targeted to youths using social media (https://www.facebook.com/Shisha-Picnic-397247207419187/photos/?ref=page_internal)

inhale more toxins than those who smoke cigarettes (Abraham et al., 2019; Martinasek et al., 2019). It stands to reason that Facebook should prohibit such adverts as *shisha* has serious consequences to people's health, particularly young people.

The shifts in marketing strategies and the development of various tobacco products are not the only changes that the tobacco industry has been making. The tobacco industry has, in recent years, vigorously targeted Africa and Asia to market their products and circumvent efforts to introduce comprehensive anti-tobacco policy and legislation (Achia, 2015;

Doku, 2010). It has been projected that tobacco advertising and promotion will further increase tobacco product use in Africa (Husain et al., 2016). However, advertising of tobacco started long back and was rife even in the USA as the case study below portrays.

Case Study 6.1: How the Industry Used Health Professionals to Influence Consumer Safety Perceptions of Cigarettes
American Tobacco became the first to use doctors/physicians in their advertisements to advance its brand "Lucky Strike", which dominated the late 1920s. The well-thought campaigns are believed to have influenced the prominence of brands such as Lucky Strikes. Company presidents worked with prominent advertising agents to develop the "reason why" consumers should opt for their brands. Even though there was no evidence to prove their claims, American Tobacco deceived the public claiming that the "toasting" process Lucky Strikes tobacco decreased irritation of the throat. These claims were unfounded and, the product curing process did not improve the safety of the product as claimed, nor did it make the brand different from the rest. Furthermore, consumers, particularly women, were persuaded to smoke "Luckies" to help them stay slim ("Reach for a Lucky instead of a sweet"). An example of the advert would read, "20,679 Physicians say 'LUCKIES are less irritating'", showing endorsements by Physicians. Adapted from (Gardner & Brandt, 2006).

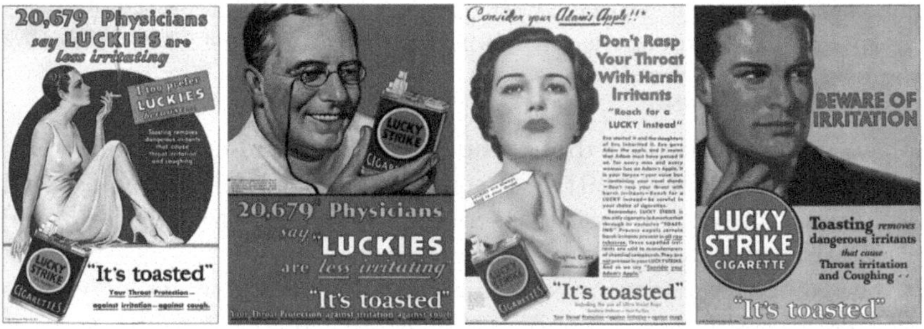

Fig. 6.3 Images of adverts on "Luckies" portraying the safety of the products on the throat and endorsements by Physicians (Gardner & Brandt, 2006)

Stop and Reflect

1. Discuss the merits or demerits of the above case study.
2. What impact can the above case study and the images shown have on smoking initiation, especially among youth and women?
3. Discuss how the tobacco industry has used influential people in your country to advance certain tobacco brands?
4. Discuss any strategies that you think the tobacco industry uses to attract women and young girls to smoking?
5. Why is the consumption of tobacco shifting from developed to developing countries?

In light of these findings, policies on tobacco advertising ought to address not only the traditional tobacco products but also new and emerging tobacco products such as e-cigarettes, vapes and *shisha* as the public mistakenly considers them to be healthier alternatives to traditional cigarette smoking (Kahr et al., 2015; Rahman et al., 2014). Additionally, countries in sub-Saharan Africa would have to address the industry's intensified marketing strategies and efforts that undermine policies designed to protect the public from tobacco products.

Global Response to the Tobacco Industry's Interference and Advertising

In response to the tobacco epidemic, the WHO adopted its Framework Convention on Tobacco Control (WHO FCTC) in 2003. The WHO FCTC comprises 38 articles on tobacco control (see WHO, 2005), but this chapter will focus on *Article 5.3* (measures to prevent tobacco industry interference on public health policies) and *Article 13* (tobacco advertising, promotion, and sponsorship). These two articles have catalysed strong tobacco control policies and strategies that reject industry interference in public health policy and its advertising efforts, particularly in high-income countries. As a result, tobacco consumption rates have dropped drastically over the past 20 years in most high-income countries such as the USA, Australia, Britain, and most European countries (WHO, 2019). However, tobacco consumption has increased to unprecedented levels in LMICs, especially in Asia and Africa (WHO, 2019). The tobacco industry has, in recent years, vigorously targeted Africa and Asia to market their products and circumvent the efforts to introduce comprehensive FCTC compliant legislation (Doku, 2010). Should Articles 5.3 and 13 be comprehensively implemented across sub-Saharan Africa, similar results could be expected. *Article 5.3* is elaborated below.

Article 5.3: Measures to Prevent Tobacco Industry Interference in Public Health Policies

The tobacco industry has employed several tactics to derail government efforts to control tobacco. Some of the tactics include "manoeuvering to hijack the political and legislative processes; exaggerating the economic importance of the industry; manipulating public opinion to gain the appearance of respectability; fabricating support through front groups; discrediting proven science; and intimidating governments with litigation or the threat of litigation" (WHO, 2012, p. 8). It is against this backdrop that *Article 5.3* of the WHO FCTC was adopted and the guidelines for its implementation developed (WHO, 2012). Embedded in the guidelines is the duty of governments to stop tobacco industry interference. In Kenya, for example, the tobacco industry interfered with Kenya's tobacco control policies. The Tobacco Control Act took nearly 13 years to go through parliament before it was finally passed and enacted into law in 2007. This was due to the industry's manipulation of the parliamentarians, including providing lavish holidays in the guise of building their capacity on the legislation (Government of Kenya, 2013).

Parties to the convention are required to develop policies that will comprehensively restrict government interactions with the tobacco industry, prohibit voluntary contributions from the tobacco industry, and incentives or privileges for the tobacco businesses, among others (WHO, 2018). Case Study 6.2 presents key principles of *Article 5.3*.

Case Study 6.2: The Guiding Principles of Article 5.3

(a) Irreconcilable conflicts exist between the interest of the tobacco industry and public health policy
(b) There is a need for transparency and accountability from all parties when addressing the tobacco industry and its interests
(c) The tobacco industry should operate and act in an accountable and transparent manner
(d) There should be no support or incentives that enable the tobacco industry to establish or run their businesses as their products are harmful and lethal to the population.

Adapted from WHO (2012, p. 15).

Stop and Reflect

1. Discuss the meaning of "irreconcilable conflict between the tobacco industry's interests and public health policy interests".
2. Why should countries require the tobacco industry and those working to further its interests to declare their interests?
3. Tobacco products are legal in most countries; however, *Article 5.3* requires that the tobacco industry, unlike other industries, should not be granted incentives to run their businesses. Discuss the possible reasons behind the non-granting of incentives.

The principles behind Article 13 are highlighted below and some success stories of countries that have implemented the guidelines for tobacco advertising, promotion and sponsorships (TAPS) in order to effectively reduce the sale and consumption of tobacco products are shared.

Article 13: Tobacco Advertising, Promotion, and Sponsorship (TAPS)

The WHO FCTC (WHO, 2005, p. 4) defines tobacco advertising and promotion as "any form of commercial communication, recommendation or action with the aim, effect or likely effect of promoting a tobacco product or tobacco use either directly or indirectly". On the other hand, tobacco sponsorship refers to "any form of contribution to any event, activity or individual with the aim, effect or likely effect of promoting a tobacco product or tobacco use either directly or indirectly". The rationale behind *Article 13* and its implementation guidelines is to offer a course of action against TAPS by the tobacco industry (WHO, 2008). There is compelling evidence that TAPS increase tobacco use. Comprehensive bans on TAPS have been proven to decrease tobacco use (WHO 2009). According to WHO (2009), policies on TAPS should comprehensively ban all forms (direct or indirect) of TAPS, without exemption for efficacy. Parties to the convention are also required to prohibit acts that aim to promote tobacco products including acts likely to have promotional effects among others.

There have been success stories in some countries (e.g., South Africa) that have implemented the guidelines for TAPS to effectively reduce the sale and consumption of tobacco products (McLeod-English et al., 2016). To be effective, policies on TAPS should comprehensively ban: "(1) all advertising and promotion, as well as sponsorship, without exemption, (2) direct and indirect advertising, promotion and sponsorship, (3) acts that aim at promotion and acts that have or are likely to have a promotional effect, (4) promotion of tobacco products and the use of tobacco, (5) commercial communications and commercial recommendations and actions, (6) contribution of any kind to any event, activity or individual, (7) advertising and promotion of tobacco brand names and all corporate promotion, and (8) traditional media (print, television and radio) and all media platforms, including the Internet, mobile telephones and other new technologies as well as films" (WHO, 2013, p. 31). Uganda is another success story.

Case Study 6.3: Uganda Passes FCTC Article 13 Compliant Law

In 2015, the Parliament of Uganda passed its new Tobacco Control Law with provisions on a comprehensive ban on tobacco advertising, promotion and sponsorship. The new law prohibits point of sale advertising and promotion as well as requiring pictorial health warnings covering 65% of all display areas of a tobacco pack. Supplying toys or sweets or other non-tobacco products that look like tobacco products is banned. Any communication through audio/visual means is also prohibited. The law also prohibits Government officials who are involved in the formulation of public health policies to interact with the tobacco industry and prescribes imprisonment for any official who does not comply with the requirement (Republic of Uganda, 2015).

Stop and Reflect

1. Do you think the provisions in this Act comprehensively ban TAPS?
2. Discuss the reasons for your answer above in line with the principles of Article 13.
3. Discuss if this law will have any impact on social media advertisements such as the ones reflected in the Figs. 6.1, 6.2, and 6.3 above.

MPOWER: A Tool to Assist Countries to Address and Implement Tobacco Control

MPOWER's objective is to monitor tobacco use prevention policies (*M*), protect people from tobacco smoke (*P*), offer help to quit tobacco use (*O*), warn people about the dangers of tobacco (*W*), enforce bans on TAPS (*E*) and raise tobacco taxes (*R*) (WHO, 2013, p. 4). MPOWER's main goal is to reduce smoking-attributable deaths (SADs) which are projected to rise to 8.3 million annually by 2030 (Mathers & Loncar, 2015, p. 2021).

There has been some success in efforts to protect people from second-hand smoke. Across WHO regions, some countries have made significant progress in decreasing tobacco smoking prevalence through tobacco policy implementation, like Australia, Denmark, Iran, Nepal, Uganda and Uruguay (Drope et al., 2018). Similarly, Senegal has successfully used mass media campaigns to increase the number of smokers who sought help with quitting smoking (Drope et al., 2018). In addition, policymakers in Mexico City successfully implemented a 100% smoke-free law in 2008 (Crosbie et al., 2011). Although the tobacco industry resisted by utilising the hospitality sector and promoting the passage of a federal law that required designated smoking areas, robust tobacco control advocacy activities for the smoke-free law led to the successful implementation of the new law in Mexico City (Crosbie et al., 2011).

In contrast, there have been some challenges in enforcing bans on TAPS. For example, in Kenya and Botswana, the tobacco industry distributes free tobacco display cabinets to street vendors so that their products are displayed in an appealing way to the youth, children, women and other vulnerable groups (Government of Kenya, 2013; Mbongwe et al., 2018). Peer (2018) gave an exposition of what needs to be done to control use of tobacco products (see Case Study 6.4 below).

Case Study 6.4: Current Strategies Are Inadequate to Curb Rising Tobacco Use

Although some African countries have achieved noteworthy success in implementing WHO FCTC articles, there is still laxity in translating this commitment into effective implementation of tobacco control and programmes. The continent also has lower rates of tobacco taxation, weaker smoke-free policies, and less restrictions on tobacco advertising when compared to other world regions. Thus, strong tobacco control policies are needed in addition to reducing tobacco industry interference through exposing the industry's misconducts where they exist. African countries need empowerment to deal with the subversive tactics of the industry, and governments need to implement and enforce effective and evidence-based tobacco control policies. Failure to do this will inevitably result in threats to public health and sustainable human development in Africa. Adapted from Peer (2018, p. 551; abstract).

Stop and Reflect

1. In your own opinion, why have African countries not been able to implement tobacco control policies as successfully as countries in the developed world have?
2. Discuss the ways in which the tobacco industry's interference and manipulation could be exposed and addressed.
3. What could you and other citizens do to influence your country's local and national politicians to implement stronger tobacco control policies?

Conclusion

In general, the WHO FCTC has played a crucial role in fast-tracking and reinforcing tobacco control measures. However, the tobacco industry's marketing strategies and interference continue to be a significant obstacle to further advancement. Selective and partial application of specific guideline recommendations in sub-Saharan Africa enables interference by the tobacco industry. In order to curb the growth of tobacco use in sub-Saharan Africa, countries in the region will have to fully commit and implement all the provisions in the WHO FCTC and MPOWER.

End of Chapter Questions

1. If you were a legislator or parliamentarian, discuss how you would protect tobacco control policies from the harmful influence of the tobacco industry using Article 5.3 in the context of your country?
2. How can cross-border advertising effectively be barred in your country if you are surrounded by countries that are not parties to the WHO FCTC?

References

Abraham, E. A., Egbe, C. O., & Ayo-Yusuf, O. A. (2019). News media coverage of shisha in Nigeria from 2014 to 2018. *Tobacco Induced Diseases, 17*, 33. https://doi.org/10.18332/tid/106139

Achia, T. N. O. (2015). Tobacco use and mass media utilisation in sub-Saharan Africa. *PLoS One, 10*(2) https://doi.org/10.1371/journal.pone.0117219

Action on Smoking and Health. (2019). *Why Big Tobacco sponsors Formula 1.* London. http://ash.org.uk/media-and-news/blog/big-tobacco-f1/. 18. Jackson J.

Britton, J. (2017). Death, disease, and tobacco. *The Lancet, 389*(10082), 1861–1862.

Crosbie, E., Sebrié, E. M., & Glantz, S. A. (2011). Strong advocacy led to the successful implementation of smoke-free Mexico city. *Tobacco Control, 20*(1), 64–72. https://doi.org/10.1136/tc.2010.037010.

Doku, D. (2010). The tobacco industry tactics-a challenge for tobacco control in low and middle-income countries. *African Health Sciences, 10*(2).

Drope, J., Schluger, N., Cahn, Z., Drope, J., Hamill, S., Islami, F., Liber, A., Nargis, N., & Stoklosa, M. (2018). *The tobacco atlas.* The American Cancer Society, and vital strategies (6th ed.). https://www.tobaccoatlas.org

Federal Trade Commission. (1986). Report to congress pursuant to the Federal Cigarette Labeling and advertising act of 1984. Federal Trade Commission.

Federal Trade Commission. (2021, March 30). *FTC releases reports on cigarette and smokeless tobacco sales and marketing expenditures for 2019.* https://www.ftc.gov/news-events/press-releases/2021/03/ftc-releases-reports-cigarette-smokeless-tobacco-sales-marketing

Gardner, M. N., & Brandt, A. M. (2006). "The doctors' choice is America's choice" the physician in US cigarette advertisements, 1930–1953. *American Journal of Public Health, 96*(2), 222–232.

Goldberg, M. E., Davis, R. M., & O'Keefe, A. M. (2006). The role of tobacco advertising and promotion: Themes employed in litigation by tobacco industry witnesses. *Tobacco Control, 15*((suppl 4), iv54–iv67.

Government of Kenya. (2013). *Tobacco industry interference in Kenya: Exposing the tactics.* Pann Printers Ltd. http://tobaccotactics.org/images/8/86/Ti_interference_in_Kenya.pdf

Husain, M. J., English, L. M., & Ramanandraibe, N. (2016). An overview of tobacco control and prevention policy status in Africa. *Preventive Medicine, 91*, S16–S22. https://doi.org/10.1016/j.ypmed.016.02.017.

Kahr, M. K., Padgett, S., Shope, C. D., Griffin, E. N., Xie, S. S., Gonzalez, P. J., Levison, J., Mastrobattista, J., Abramovici, A. R., Northrup, T. F., & Stotts, A. L. (2015). A qualitative assessment of the perceived risks of electronic cigarette and hookah use in pregnancy. *BMC Public Health, 15*(1), 1–8.

Klein, J. D., & St Clair, S. (2000). Do candy cigarettes encourage young people to smoke? *BMJ, 321*, 362–365.

Ling, P. M., Haber, L. A., & Wedl, S. (2010). Branding the rodeo: A case study of tobacco sports sponsorship. *American Journal of Public Health, 100*(1), 32–41.

Martinasek, M. P., White, R. M., Wheldon, C. W., & Gibson-Young, L. (2019). Perceptions of non-traditional tobacco products between asthmatic and non-asthmatic college students. *Journal of Asthma, 56*(5), 498–504.

Mathers, C. D., & Loncar, D. (2015). Projections of global mortality and burden of disease from 2002 to 2030. *PLoS One, 3*(11). https://doi.org/10.1371/journal.pmed.0030442.

Mbongwe, B. (2019). *Empty promises.* https://www.facebook.com/photo.php?fbid=2355926211136883&set=pb.100001585803626.-2207520000..&type=3

Mbongwe, B., Tapera, R., Katlholo, T., Erick, P., Rahube, T., Nsebula, N., Mokgethi, I., Chuma, M., Boitumelo, K., Molebatsi, M., & Tumoyagae, T. (2018). *Situational, analysis on tobacco control in Botswana.* University of Botswana (The Anti-Tobacco Network Botswana).

McLeod-English, L., Hsia, J., & Malarcher, A. (2016). Tobacco advertising, promotion, and sponsorship (TAPS) exposure, anti-TAPS policies, and students' smoking behaviour in Botswana and South Africa. *Preventive Medicine, 91*, S28–S34. https://10.1016/j.ypmed.2016.01.014

Noland, M., Ickes, M. J., Rayens, M. K., Butler, K., Wiggins, A. T., & Hahn, E. J. (2016). Social influences on use of cigarettes, e-cigarettes, and hookah by college students. *Journal of American College Health, 64*(4), 319–328.

Patel, P., Okechukwu, C. A., Collin, J., & Hughes, B. (2009). Bringing 'Light, Life & Happiness': British American Tobacco and music sponsorship in sub-Saharan Africa. *Third World Quarterly, 30*(4). https://doi.org/10.1080/01436590902867110.

Peer, N. (2018). Current strategies are inadequate to curb the rise of tobacco use in Africa. *South African Medical Journal, 108*(7), 551–556.

Rahman, S., Chang, L., Hadgu, S., Salinas-Miranda, A. A., & Corvin, J. (2014). Prevalence, knowledge, and practices of hookah smoking among university students. *Preventing Chronic Disease, 11.*

Republic of Uganda. (2015). *The tobacco control act, 2015.* https://health.go.ug/sites/default/files/Uganda_Tobacco_Control_Act_0.pdf

Stroud, L. R., Papandonatos, G. D., Borba, K., Kehoe, T., & Scott-Sheldon, L. (2019). Flavored electronic cigarette use, preferences, and perceptions in pregnant mothers: A correspondence analysis approach. *Addictive Behaviors, 91*, 21–29. https://doi.org/10.1016/j.addbeh.2018.10.043

Vasiljevic, M., Petrescu, D. C., & Marteau, T. M. (2016). Impact of advertisements promoting candy-like flavoured e-cigarettes on appeal of tobacco smoking among children: An experimental study. *Tobacco Control, 25*(e2), e107–e112.

Vice J. (2012). *Media attacked for making tobacco adverts for Philip Morris.* London. Accesses https://www.theguardian.com/media/2016/mar/17/vice-media-attacked-formaking-tobacco-adverts-for-philip-morris.

White, C., Oliffe, J. L., & Bottorff, J. L. (2012). From the physician to the Marlboro Man: Masculinity, health, and cigarette advertising in America, 1946–1964. *Men and Masculinities, 15*(5), 526–547. https://doi.org/10.1177/1097184X12461917.

World Health Organization. (2005). *WHO framework convention on tobacco control.* World Health Organization. https://www.who.int/tobacco/framework/WHO_FCTC_english.pdf

World Health Organization. (2008). *Guidelines for implementation of article 5.3 of the WHO framework convention on tobacco control.* World Health Organization. www.who.int/fctc/guidelines/adopted/article_5_3/en/

World Health Organization. (2009). *WHO report on the global tobacco epidemic: Implementing smoke-free environments.* World Health Organization. https://www.who.int/publications/i/item/9789241563918

World Health Organization. (2012). *Tobacco industry interference: A global brief.* World Health Organization. https://apps.who.int/iris/bitstream/handle/10665/70894/WHO_NMH_TFI_12.1_eng.pdf?sequence=1&isAllowed=y

World Health Organization. (2013). *WHO framework convention on tobacco control: Guidelines for implementation of article 5. 3, articles 8 to 14.* World Health Organization.

World Health Organisation. (2018). *Good country practices in the implementation of WHO FCTC Article 5.3 and its guidelines.* World Health Organisation. https://www.who.int/fctc/publications/fctc-article-5-3-best-practices.pdf

World Health Organisation. (2019). *WHO global report on trends in prevalence of tobacco use 2000–2025.* World Health Organisation. https://www.who.int/publications/i/item/who-global-report-on-trends-in-prevalence-of-tobacco-use-2000-2025-third-edition

CHAPTER 7

Impact of Illicit Substances on Health

Tshephiso Theodora Khame and Magen Mhaka-Mutepfa

Abstract Despite the four categorized key groups of substances namely, stimulants (e.g., cocaine), depressants (e.g., alcohol), opium-related painkillers (e.g., heroin), and hallucinogens (e.g., LSD), there are a few other substances that do not fit into any particular category (e.g., caffeinated energy drink). While tobacco and alcohol are the most common forms of substances known for the harms they cause to human health, there are other equally illicit harmful substances that have deleterious effects on health. These include psychoactive substances (e.g., marijuana), amphetamine-type stimulants (e.g., ecstasy, amphetamines, and methamphetamine), opiates (e.g., heroin), and stimulants (e.g., cocaine and "khat"). The aforementioned illicit substances will be discussed in this chapter. While there is indisputable evidence that substance use causes heart disease, cancer, and other non-communicable diseases, there is anecdotal evidence on the influence of illicit drugs on health (e.g., the less common drugs). The impact of illicit substances on health and wellbeing

T. T. Khame • M. Mhaka-Mutepfa (✉)
Department of Psychology, Faculty of Social Sciences, University of Botswana, Gaborone, Botswana
e-mail: khamet@ub.ac.bw; mutepfam@ub.ac.bw

M. Mhaka-Mutepfa (ed.), *Substance Use and Misuse in sub-Saharan Africa*, https://doi.org/10.1007/978-3-030-85732-5_7

and factors that lead to the use of illicit substances are also discussed. The effects that each substance has on the physical and mental health of individuals and communities are also debated, including resultant diseases. The early signs of diseases due to substance use are detected late, making it difficult to intervene timeously. Lastly, a brief evidence of intervention is presented.

Keywords Illicit drugs • Harmful impact • Physical and mental health • Substance use disorders • Resultant diseases • Transit routes

Introduction

"Health is a state of complete physical, mental, and social well-being and not merely the absence of disease or infirmity" (WHO, 2021, p. 100). Substance use is associated with a wide range of health and social problems in many instances, thereby impacting people's quality of life (QOL) and wellbeing. Illicit substance use is a major public health problem worldwide (Kavak et al., 2019) and is associated with an increased number of negative health outcomes. Physical health complications from substance use have been known to include heart disease, stroke, hypertension, sexual assault and rape, unintended pregnancies, and unintentional fatal accidents following substance use (Olawole-Isaac et al., 2018). Substance use is also associated with mental health issues, for example, using "khat" has been linked to the onset of psychosis (Ongeri et al., 2019).

Over the years, the use of illicit drugs has increased in the world including in Africa, where alarmingly children have been reported to also partake in the consumption of these substances (Fernandes & Mokwena, 2020; Odejide, 2006). The consumption of psychoactive substances such as marijuana is a practice entrenched in most African societies as it has been used for rituals, medical, ceremonial, and recreational purposes since time immemorial (International Drug Policy Consortium [IDPC], 2021). Nonetheless, an increase in illicit drug use in sub-Saharan Africa has only been noticed since 2005 (Odejide, 2006). Recently, there has been increased production and smuggling of illegal substances in Africa which include heroin, cocaine, and amphetamine-type stimulants (ATS) (IDPC, 2021). This has the potential to negatively impact the overall physical and mental health of individuals and communities.

The impact of tobacco use on health has been discussed in detail in Chap. 5 and the impact of alcohol on health has been discussed in Chap. 3. It should be noted that marijuana is used as both an illicit (e.g., Benin and Botswana) and licit substance (e.g., Zambia, Lesotho, Zimbabwe, and Malawi), depending on the legislation in different countries. The use and impact of marijuana, amphetamine-type stimulants (ATS), "khat", heroin, cocaine, and whoonga on health will be discussed below.

Use and Impact of Marijuana (Cannabis) as a Psychoactive Substance

Marijuana has been used for medicinal and traditional purposes since the nineteenth century (Owen et al., 2013). Marijuana is also known as cannabis, pot, weed, or dagga. It is perhaps the most widely used illicit substance in the African region, with the highest prevalence (5.2%–13.5%) in West and Central Africa (WHO, 2021). Evidence suggests that marijuana is used to reduce stress or trauma, especially among refugees in Mozambique, Uganda, Democratic Republic of Congo (DRC), and other war-laden countries mostly during and after the civil wars (Odejide, 2006). Marijuana is said to possess beneficial medicinal effects because it has cancer-fighting properties and is used in the treatment of autoimmune diseases (Owen et al., 2013).

Despite the aforementioned beneficial medicinal qualities, negative effects of consuming marijuana have been noted. Marijuana smoke contains similar components as those found in tobacco smoke despite not having nicotine, thus it produces similar complications related to tobacco use which have been described in detail in Chap. 5. Daily marijuana smoking has been shown to increase the risk for pulmonary symptoms such as wheezing, coughing, and sputum production (Owen et al., 2013) as well as other respiratory complications including chronic bronchitis and chronic obstructive pulmonary disease (COPD). Marijuana has also been associated with mental health-related behaviours like anxiety, suicidal behaviour, loneliness, and risky sexual behaviours (Asante, 2019).

Previous studies on marijuana and mental health effects found an association between marijuana use and the onset of psychosis (e.g., schizophrenia) (e.g., Degenhardt et al., 2013; Foti et al., 2010). In addition, Foti et al. (2010) found that those that continued to use marijuana following the onset of psychosis experienced more severe symptoms down the line. The substance has also become popular among young people, with 15.65% of adolescents in sub-Saharan Africa reportedly using it

(Olawole-Isaac et al., 2018). This may lead to long-term use and dependence (Manu et al., 2020). Thus, there is need for urgent intervention.

Use and Impact of Amphetamine-type Stimulants (ATS)

ATS, such as ecstasy and methamphetamine, are some of the substances that have been discovered mostly in sub-Saharan Africa and elsewhere (IDPC, 2021). These drugs are mostly produced in North Africa, some West African countries (e.g., Nigeria), and South Africa (IDPC, 2021). ATS has street names including ice, meth, crystal, crank, bennies, and speed and in South Africa, crystal methamphetamine in particular is called tik (Asante & Lentoor, 2017). Students believe that ATS improve intellectual performance, so they use them to stay awake and study (Cropsey et al., 2017). In addition, school environmental factors such as bullying and physical violence have been highlighted to be related to amphetamine use among school-going adolescents in Ghana (Asante, 2019). The same study also noted personal factors such as absconding from lessons, smoking, and parental substance use to predict lifetime use of amphetamine.

This is particularly distressing because not only will these students develop a lifetime dependency on the substance but will also endure harmful effects such as depression, hallucinations, aggressive behaviours, and in extreme cases, methamphetamine-induced psychosis, increasing the global burden of disease of the substance. Amphetamine use has also been associated with similar negative mental health related outcomes to marijuana, specifically loneliness and suicide behaviours (Asante, 2019).

Case Study 7.1: Ice at Its Best

"Man oh man, never take ice!!! This drug makes you do things you have never done before. If it tells you to kill a person, you kill a person. If it tells you to go on top of a moving vehicle you do exactly that. The things I did when I used to take ice, you don't want to know. I tried killing myself several times, and I had sex with whoever was available without protection. Even after quitting, my QOL and wellbeing has been affected because I…my wife left me, I contracted HIV and so did two out of my five children. Man ohh man! I will never ever do ice again neither will I do any substance."

(M. Mutepfa, personal communication, June 28, 2019)

Stop and Reflect

1. Discuss other negative effects of ice you have seen or heard about.
2. What is your take on this case? Discuss.
3. What advice would you give to substance users in your cohort?
4. What are the possible public health interventions that can be instituted to reduce the use of these substances?

Use and Impact of "Khat" (*Catha edulis*) as a Stimulant

"Khat" has been grown in Africa since the nineteenth century and has many names, depending on the region (e.g., "***miraa***", ***mairungi, cat, and Catha***) (Hartney, 2020). "Khat" leaves (which can be made into tea) contain alkaloids and are structurally related to amphetamines (Gebremedhin et al., 2013). The plants' leaves, buds, or stalks are chewed until a juice is released, which is then swallowed by the user for the pleasurable, stimulating effect (Orlien et al., 2018). Initially, "khat" was restricted to older members of the Muslim communities. However, its use has spread to many other age groups and social settings, especially in countries such as Ethiopia (Economic Botany, 1973 as cited in Gebremedhin et al., 2013). It is used during various settings such as weddings, funerals, and for recreation (Berhane et al., 2019). Its uses and health consequences are similar to ATS especially psychosis (Odenwald et al., 2005). However, its effects do not last long. The user has to continuously consume this plant in order to maintain the effects, resulting in prolonged use. Prolonged use could cause additional physical health complications including but not limited to liver disease, mouth cancer, fertility problems, and/or sleep-related issues (Elbendary et al., 2020; Orlien et al., 2018).

Use and Impact of Heroin as an Opium-Related Pain Killer

Heroin is one of the substances that was introduced into Africa due to the transit routes from South America to Europe (IDPC, 2021). The consumption of this substance seems to be concentrated along the East African coast (particularly in Kenya, Mauritius, Seychelles, and the United Republic of Tanzania) (IDPC, 2021). Heroin is largely consumed by youths in Africa (IDPC, 2021). It is smoked either with cigarettes, marijuana, or as fumes through what is referred to as "chasing the dragon" (heating heroin over a piece of foil and inhaling the vapour) (Morgan, Daniels, et al., 2019; Odejide, 2006) and is also injected, perpetuating the spread of blood-borne diseases like HIV and hepatitis (Tavitian-Exley et al., 2015). Users share needles and do not sterilize them (Atkinson et al., 2011). The aforementioned authors studied 298 young heroin injectors (17–25-year-olds) and 22% used needles that had been used by others for up to 30 days. The youths were also more prone to have more sexual partners and trade sex for money, especially among women (Atkinson et al., 2011), putting them at higher risk of contracting sexually transmitted infections (STIs). Women were also exposed to other harmful conditions like violence (Kurth et al., 2018), impacting their physical and mental wellbeing.

Physically, people who inject heroin tend to use needles which are too large to be inserted into small veins and so damage to veins has been a common phenomenon amongst people who inject drugs (PWID) (Beckerleg et al., 2005). Heroin users are also more at risk of developing physical ailments such as arthritis, hypertension, heart conditions, diabetes, and abnormal blood glucose levels, especially as they become older (Rosen et al., 2011). With respect to mental health, users had higher prevalence of lifetime post-traumatic stress disorder (PTSD), major depression, anxiety, and other mood disorders (Morgan, William, et al., 2019). Heroine also has high dependence levels (Atkinson et al., 2011), making it difficult to quit. Thus, the likelihood of people staying dependent on heroin as they age is quite high. In fact, to some, heroin dependence is characterized as a lifelong illness (Rosen et al., 2011).

Case Study 7.2: "We Can't Quit"

University students aged 18 and 19 years were on heroine; they had been injecting it for the past year. At first they used the upkeep money they would get from their parents. As their need for more doses grew, the less the few shillings they were given sufficed. They began to turn to performing sexual favours and stealing from classmates to support their habit. When asked why they would go to these extreme lengths instead of just stopping, all they could say was "We can't quit". They expressed that even though they have tried, the withdrawal symptoms were just too much to handle. The constant pain, nausea, and cold sweats became unbearable, thus resulting in a relapse. "It felt so good to have it again" they recalled, "We felt at ease again. I don't think we can quit".

(T. Khame, personal communication, February 20, 2021)

Stop and Reflect

1. Discuss the possible risks the students and the people around them may face in future.
2. Medical detox has been proven to help users successfully cease the use of heroin. Discuss any medical centres locally or in sub-Saharan Africa that have rehabilitation programmes. What are their success rates?
3. How did the two girls end up dependent on heroine? Discuss theories associated with learning new habits with regard to substance use.

Use and Impact of Cocaine

Cocaine has become one of the most commonly sniffed and smoked illicit substances in Africa in recent years, with a high prevalence in West and Central Africa as well as Southern Africa (IDPC, 2021). Cocaine is used for its stimulating effects such as enhancing alertness and giving a feeling of euphoria (Peacock et al., 2020) and can cause psychosis and paranoia. Cocaine can also cause dependence following recurrent use and subsequently cause death at high doses. It is also known to have been used by great minds such as Albert Einstein and Sigmund Freud (Oliver, 2017), which can lead to modelling and social learning as they were revered individuals. The proportion of cocaine use among adolescents in sub-Saharan Africa has been reported to be at 41.6%, with the highest proportion being in Southern Africa (Olawole-Isaac et al., 2018). Cocaine consumption started mostly because countries like Nigeria and South Africa were used as transit hubs (IDPC, 2021). These routes can be seen in Fig. 7.1 below.

With the regular use of the substance, there comes the risk of adverse health effects. With the increase in alertness comes an increase in blood pressure and heart rate, which in the long run could lead to cardiovascular complications such as stroke and arrhythmia, psychotic episodes, and suicidal ideation (Peacock et al., 2020). How cocaine is consumed can also affect the severity of these health outcomes. Smoking cocaine has been associated with respiratory problems; snorting cocaine with nasal ulcerations; and injecting cocaine leads to the increase of blood-borne virus transmission and acquisition (see Peacock et al., 2020, p. 426). Injecting substances has proven to be a factor in the spread and severity of outcomes such as HIV (Tavitian-Exley et al., 2015).

The crack form of cocaine has also been found to be a factor of the risk of dependence. Individuals who consume the crack form (crystal/

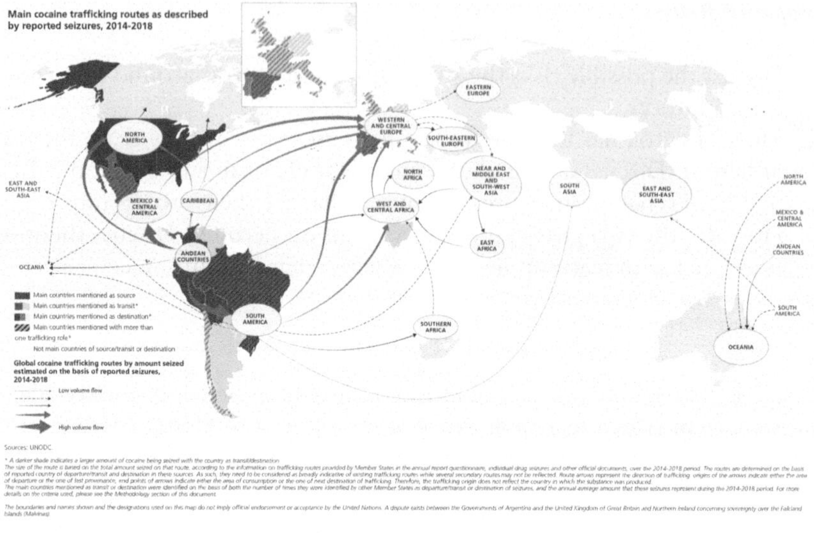

Fig. 7.1 Illustration of the flow of cocaine through West Africa and South Africa in 2014–2018 (United Nations Office on Drugs and Crime (UNODC), 2020)

rock-like appearance and of typically higher purity) are at a higher risk of developing dependence to the drug as compared to individuals who use it in the powder form (Peacock et al., 2020). It has been suggested that people with regular or problematic use of cocaine, on average, have six times greater mortality rate than their age-matched counterparts due to drug-related or traumatic causes (e.g., suicide, accidental injury, or homicide), communicable disease (e.g., AIDS-related mortality), and cardiovascular diseases (Peacock et al., 2020).

Use and Impact of Whoonga

The use of whoonga (also known as "wunga" and "nyaope"), particularly when smoked, can contribute to the spread of communicable diseases such as tuberculosis because some people smoke the same joint (Fernandes & Mokwena, 2020). Smoking whoonga, just as smoking tobacco, will likely worsen lung failure when someone contracts COVID-19 and slows the efforts of controlling the spread of the virus. Whoonga's properties and its effect on health are described in the case study below.

Case Study 7.3: "Whoonga- the Cruelest Drug of South African Slums"

'Whoonga' is a cheap, easily accessible and common deadly drug in South African slums. It is a concoction of rat poison, soap powder, and the main ingredient efavirenz found in antiretroviral (ARV) medication. Whoonga is distributed as a fine white powder that is added to marijuana or tobacco and then smoked. The mixture is highly addictive and is considered one of the most lethal drugs in the world. It "leads to violent side-effects such as anxiety, aggression, stomach cramps, and slowing of the heart rate and lungs" (Strydom, 2010, para. 3). If overdosed, the reduction in heart and lung function can become fatal. The withdrawal symptoms involve both extreme craving and pain, which are only temporarily relieved by fresh doses of the drug. A few users have allegedly died from crippling stomach cramps and acute pain as a result of withdrawal.

Its users have been known to turn to crime to feed their dependence. There have been several alarming reports indicating that patients with HIV/AIDS are being robbed of their ARVs when leaving local clinics, leading to sporadic intake or them going without their medication. Other patients are willing to sell their medication, highlighting that free ARVs are now valuable for reasons other than their intended purpose (i.e., to save lives). Corrupt health workers have also been reported to sell ARVs illegally to whoonga producers. Several users are said to intentionally seek to become HIV positive to access a steady supply of free ARVs. This is a dreadful blow in the battle against HIV and AIDS.

Whoonga has created a great deal of media attention and it is feared for its social implications. Substances used to make the mixture, such as rat poison, soap powder, and ARVs, cannot be banned because they are legal substances. South African authorities, the police, and the National Addiction Council are failing to turn the tide around because of limited resources and ignorance among its people. However, Project Whoonga (an intervention civil group), is making a difference and needs all the help it can get.

Adapted from Strydom (2010) and Mthembi et al. (2018).

Stop and Reflect

1. Discuss the economic, social, and political impacts and implications of whoonga given the growing trend of drug use in societies in sub-Saharan Africa.
2. What lessons have you learnt about using drugs such as whoonga? Discuss.
3. Discuss how you would prepare an intervention protocol to mitigate the use of whoonga.

The inclusion of ARVs into the whoonga mix brings more negative health impacts as they are not just using one substance (see the previous case study). The psychiatric side-effects that come with the ingestion of ARVs such as agitation, anxiety, hallucinations, insomnia, lethargy, nervousness, mood disorders, depression, suicidality, antisocial behaviour, psychosis, catatonia, delirium, and vivid dreams may also be problematic for whoonga users (Mthembi et al., 2018). In South Africa, the drug is mainly used by young African and coloured men (Mthembi et al., 2018), as well as young poor unemployed people in primarily Black townships (Fernandes & Mokwena, 2020). Women, including those who are pregnant, have also fallen victim to whoonga (Mthembi et al., 2018). Studies have shown that whoonga mixtures which had ARVs in them had caused complications in pregnant women such as abnormal intrauterine growth, neonatal abstinence syndrome, and abnormal behaviour for the unborn child (Mthembi et al., 2018).

The negative impacts of whoonga and other illicit substances on physical and mental health warrant timely and effective intervention to inhibit their use especially by the youth. The following section explores interventions that have been implemented.

Evidence of Interventions Used

In 2018, a study by Olawole-Isaac et al. (2018) revealed that trends of substance use among adolescents had increased, especially with cocaine, which suggested that access to these substances had gotten easier. Drug policies, such as the African Union Plan of Action on Drug Control (2013–2017), have been introduced to try and stop the growth of illicit drug use (IDPC, 2021). However, it has been noted that most of these policies led to "gross human rights violations and greater drug-related harms" (IDPC, 2021). These policies did more harm than good and were reported to have failed to make a significant reduction in the illicit market (IDPC, 2021). The IDCP (2021) attributed the failure to the policies' focus on law enforcement rather than on adopting a public health approach which would address the health harms associated with drug use and not aggravate its outcomes.

Dependence on certain drugs has been difficult to curb due to the lack of available treatment options (e.g., cocaine). Pharmacotherapies have not been found to be successful through clinical trials. Psychosocial treatment has been found to be somewhat successful in decreasing frequency of use and increasing length of abstinence. However, psychotherapy is not accessible nor affordable to most cocaine users, especially crack cocaine users as they're typically more socially marginalized (Peacock et al., 2020). Secondary interventions, which are interventions aimed at the mortality risk pathways such as HIV, could significantly aid in reducing the mortality rates but some of these are also "suboptimal" in other countries (Peacock et al., 2020).

Summary

The use of illicit substances can lead to grave psychological complications such as anxiety, depression, and paranoia. The physical effects can range from weariness and irritability to overdose, and even death. Different drugs can cause similar or different effects. Marijuana just like alcohol, impairs judgement and motor skills, and can cause damage to the lungs. Regular use of stimulants (e.g., cocaine), can lead to depression, lack of sleep, and loss of appetite. Sharing needles can spread life-threatening diseases, including AIDS, and hepatitis (a severe liver disease). Cocaine and crack claim victims from overdose, heart attack, and stroke. Heroin and other narcotics slow breathing and heart rates of users which can lead to death. Users may buy synthetic versions of street drugs which are ten times more potent than heroin and have higher risk of overdose—endangering their lives more.

Risky sexual behaviours among PWID are higher than those who do not, making users more prone to STIs and COVID-19. This was also a factor that impacted the course of the HIV/AIDS epidemic as approximately three million people with HIV/AIDS were found to partake in drug injecting (Tavitian-Exley et al., 2015). By 2018, it had been estimated that 18.7% of incident HIV infections along the Kenyan coast and 7.5% nationally had been attributed to opioid injection (Kurth et al.,

2018). Hepatitis C virus (HCV) infection has also been seen as an increasing problem particularly with PWID and TB among individuals taking heroin (Kurth et al., 2018). These risky behaviours cause a plethora of health problems and lower people's wellbeing and QOL, hence the need to intervene and prevent the use of harmful substances.

End of Chapter Questions

1. Despite their negative impact on health, ATS are also used for treating certain disorders. Discuss.
2. What are the risky behaviours that lead to people contracting communicable diseases like HIV and AIDS and COVID-19?
3. What behaviours do you personally engage in that make you more prone to use substances?
4. How can you protect yourself from becoming a victim of substance use?
5. Identify other illicit substances not mentioned in this chapter that are used in your community and negatively impact people's health.
6. How can governments put measures in place to control the use of substances?

Discussion Question

1. Discuss the different types of marijuana and the active chemicals found in the substance.

References

Asante, K. O. (2019). Cannabis and amphetamine use and its psychosocial correlates among school-going adolescents in Ghana. *Child and Adolescent Psychiatry and Mental Health, 13*(33), 33–41. https://doi.org/10.1186/s13034-019-0293-0

Asante, K. O., & Lentoor, A. G. (2017). Use of crystal methamphetamine among male adolescents in Cape Town, South Africa: Caregivers' experiences. *Substance Abuse Treatment, Prevention, and Policy, 12*(18) https://doi.org/10.1186/s13011-017-0102-9

Atkinson, J., McCurdy, S., Williams, M., Mbwambo, J., & Kilonzo, G. (2011). HIV risk behaviours, perceived severity of drug use problems and prior treatment experiences in a sample of young heroin injectors in Dar es Salaam, Tanzania. *African Journal of Drug and Alcohol Studies, 10*(1), 1–9.

Beckerleg, S., Telfer, M., & Hundt, G. L. (2005). The rise of injecting drug use in East Africa: A case study from Kenya. *Harm Reduction Journal, 2*(12) https://doi.org/10.1186/1477-7517-2-12

Berhane, Y., Canavan, C. R., Darling, A. M., Sudfeld, C. R., Vuai, S., Adanu, R., … Fawzi, W.W. (2019). The age of opportunity: Prevalence of key factors among adolescents 10-19 years of age in nine communities in sub-Saharan Africa. *Tropical Medicine and International Health, 25*(1), 15–32. https://doi.org/10.1111/tmi.13339

Cropsey, K. L., Schiavon, S., Hendricks, P. S., Froelich, M., Lentowicz, I., & Fargason, R. (2017). Mixed-amphetamine salts expectancies among college students: Is stimulant induced cognitive enhancement a placebo effect? *Drug and Alcohol Dependence, 178*, 302–309.

Degenhardt, L., Ferrari, A. J., Calabria, B., Hall, W. D., Norman, R. E., McGarth, J., & Vos, T. (2013). The global epidemiology and contribution of cannabis use and dependence to the global burden of disease: Results from the GBD 2010 study. *PLoS One, 11*(10) https://doi.org/10.1371/journal.pone.0076635

Elbendary, E. Y., Hassan, A. A., Salem, S. F., Abdalla, S. E., & Smolic, M. (2020). Prevalence and health adverse effects of 'khat' chewing among college students in Jazan region, Saudi Arabia. *Collegium Antropologicum, 44*(2), 81–86.

Fernandes, L., & Mokwena, K. E. (2020). Nyaope addiction: The despair of a lost generation. *African Journal of Drug & Alcohol Studies, 19*(1), 37–51.

Foti, D. J., Kotov, R., Guey, L. T., & Bromet, E. J. (2010). Cannabis use and the course of schizophrenia: A 10-year follow-up after first hospitalization. *American Journal of Psychiatry, 167*, 987–993.

Gebremedhin, A. T., Gesesew, H. A., Demissie, T. D., Kerie, W. M., & Sudhakar, M. (2013). 'Khat' chewing and risky sexual behaviour in sub-Saharan Africa: A systematic review protocol. *JBI Database of Systematic Reviews & Implementation Reports, 11*(12), 59–67. https://doi.org/10.11124/jbisrir-2013-877

Hartney, E. (2020, May 11). *What to know about 'khat' use*. https://www.verywellmind.com/what-is-'khat'-22092

International Drug Policy Consortium. (2021). *Policy and advocacy: Sub-Saharan Africa*. https://idpc.net/policy-advocacy/regional-work/sub-saharan-africa

Kavak, N., Çavuş, U.Y., Kavak, R.P., Sultanoğlu, H., & Doğan, B. (2019). Investigation of the clinical course and outcomes of Bonsai use. *Eurasian Journal of Emergency Medicine, 18*(2), 72–78. https://doi.org/10.4274/eajem.galenos.2019.05025.

Kurth, A. E., Cherutich, P., Conover, R., Chhun, N., Bruce, R. D., & Lambdin, B. H. (2018). The opioid epidemic in Africa and its impact. *Current Addiction Reports, 5*, 428–453. https://doi.org/10.1007/s40429-018-0232-9

Manu, E., Douglas, M., & Ayanore, M. A. (2020). Socio-ecological influences of adolescence marijuana use initiation: Qualitative evidence from two illicit marijuana-growing communities in South Africa. *South African Journal of Psychiatry, 26*(1) https://doi.org/10.4102/sajpsychiatry.v26i0.1477

Morgan, N., Daniels, W., & Subramaney, U. (2019). A prospective observational study of heroin users in Johannesburg, South Africa: Assessing psychiatric comorbidities and treatment outcomes. *Comprehensive Psychiatry*, 95. https://doi.org/10.1016/j.comppsych.2019.152137

Morgan, N., William, D., & Subramaney, U. (2019). Smoking heroin with cannabis versus injecting heroin: Unexpected impact on treatment outcomes. *Harm Reduction Journal, 16*(65) https://doi.org/10.1186/s12954-019-0337-z

Mthembi, P., Mwenesongole, E., & Cole, M. (2018). Chemical profiling of the street cocktail drug 'nyaope' in South Africa using GC-MS I: Stability studies of components of 'nyaope' in organic solvents. *Forensic Science International, 292*, 115–124. https://doi.org/10.1016/j.forsciint.2018.08.001

Odejide, A. O. (2006). Status of drug use/abuse in Africa: A review. *International Journal of Mental Health and Addiction, 4*, 87–102. https://doi.org/10.1007/s11469-006-9015-y

Odenwald, M., Neuner, F., Schauer, M., Elbert, T., Catani, C., Lingenfelder, B., Hinkel, H., Häfner, H., & Rockstroh, B. (2005). 'Khat' use as risk factor for psychotic disorders: A cross-sectional and case–control study in Somalia. *BMC Medicine, 3*(5) https://doi.org/10.1186/1741-7015-3-5

Olawole-Isaac, A., Ogundipe, O., Amoo, E. O., & Adeloye, D. (2018). Substance use among adolescents in sub-Saharan Africa: A systematic review and meta-analysis. *South African Journal of Child Health, 12*, 579–584. https://doi.org/10.7196/sajch.2018.v12i2.1524

Oliver, S. (2017, June 23). *Drugs: A brief history of Freud's love affair with cocaine*. https://www.vice.com/en/contributor/scott-oliver

Ongeri, L., Kirui, F., Muniu, E., Manduku, V., Kirumbi, L., Atwoli, L., … Mbakaya, C. (2019). 'Khat' use and psychotic symptoms in a rural 'khat' growing population in Kenya: A household survey. *BMC Psychiatry, 19*(1), 137. https://doi.org/10.1186/s12888-019-2118-3

Orlien, S. M. S., Sandven, I., Berhe, N. B., Ismael, N. Y., Ahmed, T. A., Stene-Johansen, K., Gundersen, S. G., Morgan, M. Y., & Johannessen, A. (2018). 'Khat' chewing increases the risk for developing chronic liver disease: A hospital-based case-control study. *Hepatology, 68*(1), 248–257.

Owen, K. P., Sutter, M. E., & Albertson, T. E. (2013). Marijuana: Respiratory tract effects. *Clinical Reviews in Allergy & Immunology, 46*, 65–81. https://doi.org/10.1007/s12016-013-8374-y

Peacock, A., Tran, L. T., Larney, S., Stockings, E., Santo, T., Jr., Jones, H., & Degenhardt, L. (2020). All-cause and cause-specific mortality among people with regular or problematic cocaine use: A systematic review and meta-analysis. *Society for the Study of Addiction, 116*(4), 725–742. https://doi.org/10.1111/add.15239

Rosen, D., Hunsaker, A., Albert, S. M., Cornelius, J. R., & Reynolds, C. F., III. (2011). Characteristics and consequences of heroin use among older adults in the United States: A review of the literature, treatment, implications, and recommendations for further research. *Addictive Behaviours, 36*(4), 279–285. https://doi.org/10.1016/j.addbeh.2010.12.012

Strydom, J. (2010, November 17). *Whoonga: The cruelest drug of South African slums.* https://www.globalhealth.org/whoonga-the-cruelest-drug-of-south-african-slums/

Tavitian-Exley, I., Vickerman, P., Bastos, F. I., & Boily, M.-C. (2015). Influence of different drugs on HIV risk in people who inject: Systematic review and meta-analysis. *Society for the Study of Addiction, 110*(4), 572–584. https://doi.org/10.1111/add.12846

United Nations Office on Drugs and Crime. (2020). *World drug report 2020.* United Nations Office on Drugs and Crime. https://wdr.unodc.org

World Health Organization (2021). *Substance abuse.* https://www.afro.who.int/health-topics/substance-abuse

PART II

Prevention and Intervention

CHAPTER 8

Substance Use in Organizations: Antecedents and Interventions

Mpho M. Pheko, Seth Oppong, and Leonne Mfolwe

Abstract Several micro-level factors such as substance use, about which certain workplace factors have been shown to be the precursors, can interfere with effective individual and organizational performance. Substance use is also known to lead to a vicious circle as it is related to other mental health challenges and many counterproductive work behaviours such as lateness, absenteeism, workplace incivilities as well as psychosomatic ailments and physical diseases. Accordingly, policymakers, human resources practitioners, unions and other stakeholders should take substance use seriously—whether it occurs during working hours or not. This chapter focuses on substance use in organizations and summarizes current knowledge about psychosocial factors associated with the causation and prevention of substance use within the context of organizations.

Keywords Occupational health • Workplace mental health • Workplace substance misuse • Laws and policies • Organizations • Productivity

M. M. Pheko (✉) • S. Oppong • L. Mfolwe
Department of Psychology, Faculty of Social Sciences, University of Botswana, Gaborone, Botswana
e-mail: phekom@ub.ac.bw; Oppongs@ub.ac.bw; mfolwel@ub.ac.bw

M. Mhaka-Mutepfa (ed.), *Substance Use and Misuse in sub-Saharan Africa*, https://doi.org/10.1007/978-3-030-85732-5_8

Substance Use in Organizations: Antecedents and Interventions

Organizations are open systems by their very nature, with a wide variety of factors influencing their policies, practices, processes, organizational behaviours, cultures, as well as personal and organizational outcomes (Bastedo, 2004). One of the critical resources in organizations is the human resource (Neves et al., 2013), which is impacted by an array of factors in the PESTEL (i.e., the political, economic, socio-cultural, environmental, and legislative) environments (Griffin, 2006). These factors, including the global burden of non-communicable diseases (NCDs), have heightened interests in monitoring the health, economic costs, and associated risk factors of substance use and misuse—for individuals, communities, and workplaces (Kassa & Grace, 2019). This chapter presents a summary of the literature on substance use, misuse, prevention, management, and treatment for the working population and workplaces.

It is imperative to put a spotlight on substance use and misuse for the working populations since work, working, and workplaces are central to many people's lives—with a large percentage of workers spending a greater percentage of their hours traveling to work, being at work, and commuting from work. In fact, some researchers have suggested that most users of illicit drugs and heavy drinkers are working adults (Ames & Bennett, 2011), many of whom never misused substances in adolescence (Cook & Schlenger, 2002). Given the nature of these psychoactive substances, their use and misuse may pose serious health and economic problems for the users, co-workers, and organizations. Organizations that proactively attend to substance use and possible misuse may, therefore, ensure attainment of organizational goals, sustainable growth, and demonstrate capacity for compassionate and responsive leadership; this, in turn, benefits employees, employers, shareholders, and taxpayers.

Dealing with substance use and misuse is a global concern. In 2015, the United Nations (UN) member states adopted 17 sustainable development goals (SDGs) to end poverty, protect the planet and ensure prosperity for all—which the UN member states agreed to achieve by 2030 (UN, 2016). SDG 3 seeks to ensure healthy lives and to promote well-being. It has a health target related to Target 3.5, which aims at "strengthen[ing] the prevention and treatment of substance use, including... harmful use of alcohol" (UN, 2016, p.20). The WHO (2019) further suggests that the harmful use of alcohol is one of the leading risk factors for population health worldwide and that it has a direct impact on many health-related targets of SDGs—particularly because alcohol is often consumed before, along with, or after other psychoactive substances.

Given the concerns of the UN, WHO, and the International Labour Organization (ILO) as well as the specific health, economic, and negative outcomes associated with substance use and misuse, this summary will benefit individuals studying to become researchers, policymakers, practitioners as well as other professionals such as trade unionists, human resources practitioners, safety and health experts, lawyers, medical officers, occupational health officers, and even workers themselves. Given the broadness of this topic, this chapter will mainly focus on tobacco and alcohol use and will use the phrase "substance use" to refer to both, unless otherwise stated. Additionally, the term "organization" will refer to companies of varying sizes as well as those in different sectors and industries including but not limited to the creative industry, transportation, health, and a host of related others.

Workplace Contexts and Substance Use and Misuse

Why do the working populations use and misuse substances? The sociocultural approaches, which emphasize certain aspects of the social environment (i.e., structure, social bonds, social interaction, and culture) suggest that these have an impact on each other, resulting in certain behaviour patterns. Similarly, the extant literature suggests that in workplaces, substance misuse may depend on a combination of multiple factors. Some internal (worker factors, organizational practices, polices, and cultures), and others societal (i.e., factors in the PESTEL environment). For example, Frone (2003) documented evidence that link substance use and misuse to certain socio-demographic factors, personalities, substance use outcome expectancies, substance availability, and work stressors. Prevalence also varies considerably by age group, gender, education, and occupation. Illicit drug use and/or heavy drinking is more likely to occur among young workers, males, and workers with less education, unmarried employees, and employees without children (see Thørrisen et al., 2018).

Values, Beliefs, and Attitudes: Substance Use and Misuse as a Subculture

Modelling and Normative Influence

The social learning processes (e.g., social modelling, perceived norms) and coping skills and cognitive processes (e.g., self-efficacy, outcome expectancies) asserted by Bandura (1994, 1997) can explain the processes by which social influence contributes to substance use and misuse behaviours. Modelling, which may begin with observation and imitation of substance use-specific behaviours in the environment may be socially reinforced through expectations of positive consequences from substance use, and may end with use (see Moos, 2007) or substance use disorders (SUDs). This may also explain why substance use is linked to typologies of work (e.g., rhythms, cadences, shift work), and professional natures (Buvik et al., 2018). Individuals employed as musicians and blue-collar workers tend to have preferences for different substances—even beyond alcohol and tobacco.

Case Study 8.1: Substance Misuse in the Music Industry
Brenda Fassie, a world-renowned South African popstar, led a life of substance misuse until her death in 2004. Brenda had worked in the music industry since childhood and achieved success in her early years of life. While hers is not believed to be a drug-related death, her life was characterised by substance dependence and various public scandals. A case in point was the drug-related death of her partner after they had binged on drugs together one night in 1995. The loss had deeply affected Brenda but her substance misuse had continued for years following that incident. Similar examples of accomplished musicians who battled substance dependence include Whitney Houston and Michael Jackson, both of whom died from drug overdose.

Adapted from Lategan (2004) and Walsh (2004).

Stop and Reflect

1. What work-related conditions and stressors unique to musicians can you think of?
2. How do you think that those conditions and stressors contribute to the pervasive drug use and misuse in the music industry?
3. How might Bandura's social learning processes contribute to drug use and misuse in the music industry?

Workplace Stress and Work-Family Role Strains

Maclean et al. (2015) have provided evidence linking substance use and misuse to specific work situations such as problems with co-workers, job changes, and perceived financial strain. Further, perceived self-medication benefits associated with alcohol and illicit drugs may be higher when individuals are faced with stressful workplace conditions (Maclean et al., 2015). Ames and Janes (1992) presented the alienation-stress paradigm which posits that employee alcohol use may be a response to the physical and psychosocial qualities of the work environment. Other related terms include social availability and physical availability—both of which explain substance use and misuse in working populations. Ames and Grube (1999) described *social availability* at work as the degree to which fellow workers support drinking either off or on the job, and the *physical availability* as the ease with which alcohol can be obtained for consumption on the job, during breaks, and at work-related events.

Cultural Practices and Attitudes Towards Substance Use

Social agreements and general attitudes towards substance use by the larger society have a direct impact on attitudes towards abstinence and specific substance use and misuse. This means that some factors that influence alcohol use by workers may be at the macro-level and external to the organizations but still influence alcohol consumption in the specific localities and for certain individuals. Some have linked it to the consequences of personal, family, or social factors (International Labour Organization, 1996) that may be within or outside the organization. These may include social drinking, family, and cultural practices, as well as societal views and perceptions of substance use. In some low-income countries, the use of drugs may be a normal part of the culture, affecting the supply of labour, income, consumption, and investment at the household and aggregate levels (Levy et al., 2006). Schou and Moan (2016) found the alcohol

Case Study 8.2: Alcohol Culture in Botswana
Alcohol has a firm and established place in Setswana culture. Historically, there has always been alcohol to be served at all traditional ceremonies and rituals: from weddings to initiation celebrations. Now, in recent times, its consumption has spilled over to social situations beyond traditional occasions. It, therefore, comes as no surprise that it has been found to be one of the most misused substances in Botswana.

Adapted from Sinkaba (2015).

use-sickness-absence linkages to be stronger among people with low education and low income.

Stop and Reflect

1. How does perception towards substances in your culture affect the levels of substance consumption in your community and/or organization?

Health Costs of Substance Use and Misuse

The health concerns of substance use tend to follow the **biological** and **psychological** models. This can be explained by the concern that, for some individuals, substance use can lead to substance use disorders (SUDs)—a condition in which the use of one or more substances (including psychoactive drugs such as alcohol, prescription pain medications, and marijuana) leads to a clinically significant impairment or distress (Goplerud et al., 2017). SUDs are among the most common and costly health conditions whose national costs have been estimated to exceed \$400 billion annually in the United States alone (see Tecco et al., 2013).

The most common substances are alcohol and tobacco—which tend to be viewed as less harmful than other illicit drugs. Unfortunately, these perceptions are untrue as both are amongst the leading causes of accidents and mortality (see the section on "Substance Use and Safety in the Workplace"). Both alcohol and cigarettes have strong comorbidity and dependence (WHO, 2019) and both substances are leading causes of mortality, contribute to health and economic challenges, and have been associated with significant reduction in work productivity (Suwa et al., 2017). By their nature, these two substances also have a strong negative effect on the central nervous system, impairing judgement and concentration, and putting the users, co-workers, and organizational equipment at risk.

The numbers of deaths related to tobacco use seem to be on the rise. In 2015, direct tobacco use was associated with over five million deaths annually among the estimated one billion smokers worldwide, and additional 600,000 deaths associated with second-hand smoke (Baker et al., 2017). In 2018, WHO acknowledged smoking as one of the biggest public health threats, killing more than seven million people around the world every year. First-hand smoking causes many different types of cancer, including lung, mouth, and throat cancer, and leukaemia (Troelstra et al., 2020). Therefore, smoking results in a significant societal burden that is expressible in both healthcare costs and lost productivity (Goodchild et al., 2018). However, this burden has been lessened by tobacco cessation programmes (Suwa et al., 2017). In a study to investigate the burden of smoking on productivity in the US, EU, and China, improved productivity outcomes were evident even among those who had ceased smoking relatively recently (Baker et al., 2017).

Alcohol misuse has also been identified as a major risk factor for diseases, disability, and mortality, and it has been associated with more than 200 disease and injury conditions (see World Health Organization, 2019). The leading contributors to the burden of alcohol-attributable deaths and disability-adjusted life years (DALYs) in 2016 were injuries, digestive diseases, and alcohol use disorders for men, and cardiovascular diseases, and injuries for women (World Health Organization, 2019). In one systematic review, Rehm et al. (2017) found alcohol use to be a major risk factor for disease, injuries, disability, and mortality. Because alcohol use disorders tend to be more stigmatized than even clinically severe psychiatric disorders (Schomerus et al., 2011), identifying and confronting suspicions of substance misuse can be an awkward and often complicated task, leading to possible underestimation of prevalence and impact (Rehm et al., 2017).

Job and Organizational Performance Costs of Substance Use and Misuse

Substance use and misuse may not only have an adverse effect on the health and well-being of workers but it has the potential to also lead to many work-related problems including deterioration in job performance (ILO, 1996). While the nature of the association is not always clear-cut, there has been reasonable evidence suggesting that substance use and misuse may lead to multiple negative workplace outcomes and impacts on the bottom-line through, for example, lost productivity, absenteeism, accidents, and a wide variety of other dysfunctional work behaviours (ILO, 1996).

Case Study 8.3: Alcohol and Productivity on Farms

Alcohol misuse has been linked to lessened productivity in a number of studies. A survey in South Africa revealed that the practice of offering *Dop* (cheap alcohol) to farm labourers has led to many problems on farms. Based on the results of this survey, farm labourers were more likely to be current drinkers than individuals in other occupations. Further research is needed to assess whether progressive practices on some farms will reduce harmful alcohol use.

Adapted from Gossage et al. (2014).

Stop and Reflect

1. Think of occupations and scenarios in your own locality and discuss possible prevalence, antecedents, and consequences of alcohol consumptions for each occupation and/or scenario.
2. Discuss reasons why farm workers are more likely to drink or use other harmful substances more than people in other occupations.
3. Discuss issues that emanate from the excessive drinking on farms.
4. How can stakeholders intervene to stop this harmful behaviour on farms?

Similar to alcohol, smoking can also steal from productivity. In Bunn III et al.'s (2006) study, active smokers missed more days of work and experienced more unproductive time at work compared with former smokers and non-smokers. Yet another study in the Netherlands revealed that smoking status was associated with an increased use of sick leave and lost productivity (Robroek et al., 2011). Further, Baker et al. (2017) documented evidence that active smokers reported greater absenteeism, greater presenteeism, overall work impairment, and activity impairment than former smokers and individuals who never smoked in the US, EU and China. The results further suggest that smoking cessation benefits extend to work productivity rapidly after cessation—laying a good case for the implementation of workplace substance cessation programmes (Baker et al., 2017).

According to Caulkins et al. (2014), an additional disturbing fact about substance use and misuse is that it sends hundreds of thousands of people (including workers) to medical interventions, many to jails for use and possession of illegal drugs and kills hundreds of thousands of people every year. They further state that billions of dollars in national healthcare budgets are spent on drug treatment and on treating associated medical complications and related diseases.

Substance Use and Safety in the Workplace

About half of all fatal occupational injuries are transportation-related, and the others are generally grouped into other categories of accidents such as being struck by an object or falling to a lower level (see Ramchand et al., 2009). Currently, the plethora of studies support the conclusion that alcohol and other forms of substance use are associated with higher levels of occupational injuries, whether self-reported or objective measures (Ramchand et al., 2009). Alcohol and sedative use generally lead to the suppression of the central nervous system (Ramchand et al., 2009) leading to increased reaction time, poor reasoning, poor psychomotor skills, poor exercise of caution, and poor judgement (Normand et al., 1994) and more errors. It is particularly important to also note that "substance use that occurs hours before a worker begins his or her shift can cause spillover effects, such as fatigue and hangovers that may independently increase injury risk." (Ramchand et al., 2009, p. 3). An alternative explanation for substance-related workplace injuries is that employees who misuse alcohol and other substances are also more likely to engage in other risky behaviours (Spicer et al., 2003) which negatively affects safety behaviour, whether defined as safety participation, safety compliance or both (Oppong, 2011). Noting that it takes unsafe behaviour and unsafe conditions for an accident to take place (Oppong, 2011), substance use is expected to lead to impaired decisions and poor psychomotor skills that (1) make employees fail or refuse to create safe environment for other workers through their actions and inactions (safety participation issue), (2) make them engage in unsafe or risky behaviours at work by failing to observe the safety protocols or procedures (safety compliance issue), or (3) both.

Also relevant is the fact that impaired judgement and increased reaction time have the potential to result in faculty risk perception. Substance use-risk perception-accident linkages can be examined using a theory of risk perception such as Oppong's (2011, 2015, 2021) risk chain process model. The risk chain process model holds that, among other factors, faulty risk perception results from individual factors such as decreased concentration and other cognitive impairments associated with alcohol use (Oppong, 2015, 2021). Further, the risk chain process model intimates that when employees engage in faulty risk perception, there is a higher likelihood of errors and/or risky behaviours occurring while the errors may lead to higher risk exposure with higher likelihood of accident or near misses. The impaired judgement and psychomotor skills can, through the faulty risk perception, result in any combination of the four critical errors, namely: eyes-not-on-task(s), mind-not-on-task(s), being in the line-of-fire, and poor balance/grip (see Oppong, 2011, 2015). These errors are associated with injuries, fatality, damage to properties, and/or occupational diseases.

Case Study 8.4: Flight JA 8054 Crash

A flight en-route to Tokyo from USA crashed and killed all that were on-board. Investigations determined that the crash occurred because the aircraft stalled as a result of input errors made by the pilot in an intoxicated state. A post-mortem toxicology report revealed that the pilot had a blood alcohol level of 210 mg%; levels between 180 mg% and 300 mg% have been found to cause confusion, disorientation, as well as impaired perception and coordination. The flight and the consequent crash could have also been avoided had the flight crew refused to allow the pilot to fly in his intoxicated state, which was believed to have been apparent to those that had been in contact with him that day.

Adapted from National Transportation Safety Board (1979).

Stop and Reflect

1. Can you identify the unsafe conditions and the unsafe behaviours that contributed to this accident?
2. What are the substance use-risk perception-accident linkages you can identify in the above case study through the risk chain process model?

Prevention, Management, and Treatment in Workplaces

The ILO recommends that "alcohol- and drug-related problems should be considered as health problems, and, therefore, should be dealt with, without any discrimination, like any other health problem at work and covered by the health care systems (public or private)" (ILO, 1996, p. VII). Given the multiplicity of causes of alcohol- and drug-related problems, approaches to prevention, assistance, treatment, and rehabilitation are also likely to vary (ILO, 1996)—depending on factors related to policies, regulations, laws, and personal factors.

Individuals with risky drinking habits are likely to be found in organizations (see Cook & Schlenger, 2002) because the majority of the adult population is employed. This makes the workplace an important setting for the development of substance dependence and for designing and implementing programmes and interventions for those affected by substance use and misuse (see Ames & Bennett, 2011). In essence, from the perspectives of social learning and cognitive approaches, the same factors that predispose workers to the risks of developing alcohol problems may also be the levels of change for prevention, management, and treatment of substance use and misuse in the workplaces (see Thørrisen et al., 2018). According to Bandura's (1994, 1997) social cognitive theory and its related cognitive processes that influence a person's behaviour, self-efficacy and outcome expectancies can be used to develop and enhance effectiveness, prevention and treatment programmes in organizations. Used in the context of substance use, social cognitive learning theories can explain how the processes of observing and/or imitating positive behaviours, attitudes, and models in the organizations can lead to changes in behaviour (see Giovazolias & Themeli, 2014).

Further, in line with ILO (1996) recommendations, the design of organizations presents them as platforms to ensure that information, education, and training programmes concerning alcohol and drugs are integrated into broad-based health programmes. Ames and Bennett (2011) further suggest that these programmes should be based on health promotion, social health promotion, and intervention, and even include other innovative approaches such as web-based interventions. Beyond health programmes, Ames and Bennett (2011) further suggest that employers incorporate lifestyle campaigns and encourage workers to change their individual behaviour and to identify and reduce work environment risk factors.

More concretely, strategies such as workplace drug testing, alcohol-exclusion laws, employee-assistance programmes (EAPs), education campaigns, and culture change initiatives (targeting social norms) should be used in diverse work settings (see Ramchand et al., 2009). For instance, alcohol-exclusion laws make employers non-liable to pay workers' compensation for alcohol-induced injuries, thereby shifting the responsibility to employees. While EAPs are created to offer "short-term counselling and long-term referrals to employees with emotional and behavioural concerns, including substance-use problems" (Ramchand et al., 2009, p.28), more could be achieved. For example, health education programmes could also be implemented to create awareness about the dangers of substance use and encourage self-referrals to the EAPs. Lastly, workplace substance use norms could be influenced through organizational culture change initiatives supported by "managerial structures and health-promotion and wellness programming" (Ramchand et al., 2009, p. 29).

End of Chapter Questions

1. Given the UN and the WHO's concern about prevention and treatment of substance use and misuse, what can member states and organizations in the African context do to ensure attainment of the SDG 3, Target 3.5?
2. How can the trade unions and workers benefit from knowledge about substance use, misuse, prevention, management, and treatment?
3. Given that some aspects of the work environment have been linked to substance use and misuse, should organizations and management be liable in such scenarios? Explain.
4. Reflect on alcohol consumption in your organization and think of an appropriate substance use intervention programme that uses Bandura's social cognitive theory. What features will it have? How will you ensure effectiveness of the programme?

References

Ames, G. M., & Bennett, J. B. (2011). Prevention interventions of alcohol problems in the workplace: A review and guiding framework. *Alcohol Research & Health, 34*(2), 175.

Ames, G. M., & Grube, J. W. (1999). Alcohol availability and workplace drinking: Mixed method analyses. *Journal of Studies on Alcohol, 60*(3), 383–393. https://doi.org/10.15288/jsa.1999.60.383

Ames, G. M., & Janes, C. (1992). A cultural approach to conceptualizing alcohol and the workplace. *Alcohol Research, 16*(2), 112–119. https://search.proquest.com/scholarly-journals/cultural-approach-conceptualizing-alcohol/docview/222379181/se-2?accountid=1549

Baker, C. L., Flores, N. M., Zou, K. H., Bruno, M., & Harrison, V. J. (2017). Benefits of quitting smoking on work productivity and activity impairment in the United States, the European Union and China. *International Journal of Clinical Practice, 71*(1), 1–10, e12900. https://doi.org/10.1111/ijcp.12900

Bandura, A. (1994). Self-efficacy. In V. S. Ramachaudran (Ed.), *Encyclopedia of human behavior* (Vol. 4, pp. 71–81). Academic Press.

Bandura, A. (1997). *Self-efficacy: The exercise of control*. Freeman.

Bastedo, M. N. (2004). Open systems theory. *The SAGE Encyclopedia of Educational Leadership and Administration*. http://www-personal.umich.edu/~bastedo/papers/bastedo.opensystems.pdf

Bunn, W. B., III, Stave, G. M., Downs, K. E., Alvir, J. M. J., & Dirani, R. (2006). Effect of smoking status on productivity loss. *Journal of Occupational and Environmental Medicine, 48*(10), 1099–1108. https://doi.org/10.1097/01.jom.0000243406.08419.74.

Buvik, K., Moan, I. S., & Halkjelsvik, T. (2018). Alcohol-related absence and presenteeism: Beyond productivity loss. *International Journal of Drug Policy, 58*, 71–77. https://doi.org/10.1016/j.drugpo.2018.05.005.

Caulkins, J. P., Kasunic, A., & Lee, M. A. C. (2014). Societal burden of substance abuse. *International Public Health Journal, 6*(3), 269–282.

Cook, R., & Schlenger, W. (2002). Prevention of substance abuse in the workplace: Review of research on the delivery of services. *Journal of Primary Prevention, 23*(1), 115–142.

Frone, M. R. (2003). Predictors of overall and on-the-job substance use among young workers. *Journal of Occupational Health Psychology, 8*(1), 39–54. https://doi.org/10.1037/1076-8998.8.1.39.

Giovazolias, T., & Themeli, O. (2014). Social learning conceptualization for substance abuse: Implications for therapeutic interventions. *The European Journal of Counselling Psychology, 3*(1), 69–88. https://doi.org/10.5964/ejcop.v3i1.23

Goodchild, M., Nargis, N., & d'Espaignet, E. T. (2018). Global economic cost of smoking-attributable diseases. *Tobacco Control, 27*(1), 58–64. https://doi.org/10.1136/tobaccocontrol-2016-053305

Goplerud, E., Hodge, S., & Benham, T. A. (2017). Substance use cost calculator for US employers with an emphasis on prescription pain medication misuse. *Journal of Occupational and Environmental Medicine, 59*(11), 1063–1071. https://doi.org/10.1097/JOM.0000000000001157.

Gossage, J. P., Snell, C. L., Parry, C. D. H., Marais, A., Barnard, R., de Vries, M., Blankenskip, J., Seedat, S., Hasken, J. M., & May, P. A. (2014). Alcohol use, working conditions, job benefits, and the legacy of the "Dop" system among farm workers in the Western Cape Province, South Africa: Hope despite high levels of risky drinking. *International Journal of Environmental Research and Public Health, 11*(7), 7406–7424. https://doi.org/10.3390/ijerph110707406.

Griffin, R. W. (2006). *Fundamentals of management* (4th ed.). Houghton Mifflin Company.

International Labour Organization. (1996). *Management of alcohol and drug-related issues in the workplace: An ILO code of practice.* International Labour Office.. https://www.ilo.org/public/libdoc/ilo/1996/96B09_297_engl.pdf

Kassa, M., & Grace, J. (2019). *The global burden and perspectives on non-communicable diseases (NCDs) and the prevention, data availability and systems approach of NCDs in low-resource countries.* IntechOpen. https://doi.org/10.5772/intechopen.89516

Lategan, A. (2004, May 18). *The life of Brenda Fassie.* https://www.news24.com/w24/SelfCare/Wellness/Body/The-life-of-Brenda-Fassie-20040518

Levy, A., Neri, F., & Grass, D. (2006). Macroeconomic aspects of substance abuse: Diffusion, productivity and optimal control. *Macroeconomic Dynamics, 10*, 145–164. https://doi.org/10.1017.S1365100506050140

Maclean, J. C., Webber, D., & French, M. T. (2015). Workplace problems, mental health and substance use. *Applied Economics, 47*(9), 883–905. https://doi.org/10.1080/00036846.2014.982856.

Moos, R. H. (2007). Theory-based active ingredients of effective treatments for substance use disorders. *Drug and Alcohol Dependence, 88*(2-3), 109–121.

National Transportation Safety Board. (1979). *Japan Air Lines Co., Ltd. McDonnell-Douglas DC-8-62F, JA 8054, Anchorage, Alaska, January 13*, 1977. National Transportation Safety Board. https://www.fss.aero/accident-reports/dvdfiles/US/1977-01-13-US.pdf

Neves, C., Galvão, A., & Pereira, F. (2013). Guidelines in human resources management. In J. A. C. Santos, F. Perdigão, & P. Águas (Eds.), *Book of proceedings – Tourism and management studies international conference Algarve 2012* (Vol. 2, pp. 420–429). University of the Algarve.

Normand, J., Lempert, R. O., & O'Brien, C. P. (1994). *Under the influence?* National Academy Press. http://www.nap.edu/catalog/2118.html

Oppong, S. (2011). *Health & safety: Theory and practice in the oil and gas sector.* VDM Publishing House Ltd..

Oppong, S. (2015). Risk chain process model: Linking risk perception to occupational accidents. *Sigurnost, 57*(1), 25–34.

Oppong, S. (2021). From risk perception to accident: An empirical test of the risk chain process model. *Sigurnost, 63*(2), 125–142.

Ramchand, R., Pomeroy, A., & Arkes, J. (2009). *The effects of substance use on workplace injuries.* RAND Corporation.

Rehm, J., Gmel, G. E., Sr., Gmel, G., Hasan, O. S., Imtiaz, S., Popova, S., Probst, C., Roerecke, M., Room, R., Samokhvalov, A. V., Shield, K. D., & Shuper, P. A. (2017). The relationship between different dimensions of alcohol use and the burden of disease-an update. *Addiction, 112*(6), 968–1001. https://doi.org/10.1111/add.1375.

Robroek, S. J., van den Berg, T. I., Plat, J. F., & Burdorf, A. (2011). The role of obesity and lifestyle behaviours in a productive workforce. *Occupational and Environmental Medicine, 68*(2), 134–139. https://doi.org/10.1136/oem.2010.055962.

Schomerus, G., Lucht, M., Holzinger, A., Matschinger, H., Carta, M. G., & Angermeyer, M. C. (2011). The stigma of alcohol dependence compared with other mental disorders: A review of population studies. *Alcohol and Alcoholism, 46*(2), 105–112.

Schou, L., & Moan, I. S. (2016). Alcohol use–sickness absence association and the moderating role of gender and socioeconomic status: A literature review. *Drug and Alcohol Review, 35*(2), 158–169. https://doi.org/10.1111/dar.12278.

Sinkaba, R. P. (2015). Alcohol abuse and intervention strategies in Botswana and China: A preliminary study. *Journal of African Studies, 29*(1), 157–170.

Spicer, R. S., Miller, T. R., & Smith, G. S. (2003). Worker substance use, workplace problems and the risk of occupational injury: A matched case-control study. *Journal of Studies on Alcohol, 64*(4), 570–578.

Suwa, K., Flores, N. M., Yoshikawa, R., Goto, R., Vietri, J., & Igarashi, A. (2017). Examining the association of smoking with work productivity and associated costs in Japan. *Journal of Medical Economics, 20*(9), 938–944. https://doi.org/10.1080/13696998.2017.1352507.

Tecco, J., Jacques, D., & Annemans, L. (2013). The cost of alcohol in the workplace in Belgium. *Psychiatria Danubia, 25*(2), S118–S123.

Thørrisen, M. M., Skogen, J. C., & Aas, R. W. (2018). The associations between employees' risky drinking and sociodemographics, and implications for intervention needs. *BMC Public Health, 18*(1), 735–744. https://doi.org/10.1186/s12889-018-5660-x.

Troelstra, S. A., Coenen, P., Boot, C. R., Harting, J., Kunst, A. E., & van der Beek, A. J. (2020). Smoking and sickness absence: A systematic review and meta-analysis. *Scandinavian Journal of Work, Environment & Health, 46*(1), 5–18. https://doi.org/10.5271/sjweh.3848.

United Nations. (2016). *Transforming our world: The 2030 agenda for sustainable development.* United Nations. https://sustainabledevelopment.un.org/content/documents/21252030%20Agenda%20for%20Sustainable%20Development%20web.pdf

Walsh, D. (2004, May 11). *South Africa mourns its pop diva Fassie.* https://www.irishtimes.com/news/south-africa-mourns-its-pop-diva-fassie-1.1139921

World Health Organization. (2019). *Global status report on alcohol and health 2018.* World Health Organization.

CHAPTER 9

Prescription Drug Misuse and Prevention in Sub-Saharan Africa

Rachel W. Kimani, Ability C. Katsidzira, and Farai A. Mhaka

Abstract Research has confirmed that the introduction of prescription drugs to Africa increased the availability and misuse of psychoactive substances, especially among adolescents and young adults. Although data on prescription drug use in sub-Saharan Africa remains scarce, emerging evidence highlights that prescription drug misuse (PDM) is a major concern. This chapter reviews the definitions of prescription drugs, PDM, and prescription drug disorders. In addition, the three most commonly misused psychoactive prescription drugs are discussed: stimulants (methamphetamine), opioids (codeine, tramadol), and central nervous system depressants (benzodiazepines, quaaludes, sleeping pills). Vulnerable populations are also discussed. Evidence-based prevention strategies and harm reduction in the region and treatment interventions for prescription drug disorders are explored.

R. W. Kimani (✉)
School of Nursing and Midwifery, The Aga Khan University, Nairobi, Kenya
e-mail: rachel.kimani@aku.edu

A. C. Katsidzira • F. A. Mhaka
Edendale Hospital, Pietermaritzburg, South Africa

M. Mhaka-Mutepfa (ed.), *Substance Use and Misuse in sub-Saharan Africa*, https://doi.org/10.1007/978-3-030-85732-5_9

Keywords Psychoactive substances • Prescription drugs • Hallucinogens • Steroid use • Prescription drug misuse • Harm reduction • Prevention and intervention

Introduction

Prescription drugs are 'legal' manufactured pharmaceutical compounds obtained using a clinician's written instruction (prescription) for a bona fide medical reason. Prescription drug misuse (PDM) and dependence are growing problems worldwide (United Nations Office of Drugs and Crime) (UNODC, 2010a). There have been advances in the manufacture of powerful medications that improve health and quality of life when used safely. However, misuse of psychoactive prescription medications can lead to adverse health consequences and dependence. Unlike illicit drugs (e.g., heroin, cocaine, and hallucinogens), prescription drugs are diverted for nonmedical use from the healthcare system, thereby straining the available resources for medical care. This chapter discusses the epidemiology of PDM in sub-Saharan Africa, major prescription drugs that are misused, and prevention and treatment strategies.

Historically, there has been a clear divide between illicit ('bad' or 'illegal') drugs and prescription ('good' or 'legal') drugs. However, these boundaries are blurred with the increased number of prescription drug overdose cases, such as those extensively reported in the North America opioid epidemic. Pharmacologically, prescription drugs used for recreational purposes generally fit into similar drug classes as illicit drugs. For example, oxycodone and tramadol fit into the same category as heroin (opiates), whereas methylphenidate and amphetamines are stimulants, which is the same category as cocaine. Therefore, pharmacological factors associated with illicit drug use apply to prescription drug use, and the expected drug effects may be the driving component in the addictive potential of misused prescription drugs. Doses of prescription drugs for recreational use tend to be higher than therapeutic doses, and administration of these drugs may also differ to achieve more intoxicating effects. Multi-drug use or co-ingestion may also result in additional drug reinforcement, increasing the risk for adverse effects (e.g., respiratory depression) and potentially increasing the addictive potential (Compton & Volkow, 2006).

The extent of PDM in sub-Saharan Africa is underestimated because a large proportion of the population obtains medications from the informal sector (e.g., drug trafficking), and estimates of the prevalence of substandard and falsified medicines are unreliable because drug monitoring systems remain inadequate (Peyraud et al., 2017; UNODC, 2015). In addition, misuse of substances and drug overdoses have historically been viewed as a law enforcement concern rather than a public health issue. Although misuse, addiction, and deaths relating to prescription drugs have increasingly been reported in the United States and other high-income countries, the extent of the problem in sub-Saharan Africa is not well known. Some African countries have provided recent data concerning PDM, but how the trends have evolved and how they compare with countries reporting high drug misuse have not yet been deciphered. Furthermore, as the region continues to grapple with high rates of HIV, prescription drug diversion and misuse have been identified as barriers to achieving and maintaining viral suppression (Chibi et al., 2020). Evidence-based medications and interventions to reduce infections and treat disorders exist but are limited in Africa (Kurth et al., 2018).

Conceptual Clarifications: PDM, Disorders, and Dependence

PDM is defined in numerous ways. However, a comprehensive way to explain PDM is the use of prescription medication without a prescription note/pad or use of these drugs in ways not intended by the prescriber (Schepis et al., 2020). Furthermore, PDM is not limited to intentional use of a medication with psychotropic properties outside of a clinician's prescription for a medical condition. It also includes using another person's medication, even if it is for the same medical condition, or using greater amounts of the medication, more often or for longer than intended by the prescriber (Compton & Volkow, 2006). For example, a doctor prescribes lorazepam (an intermediate-acting psycholeptic drug) for short-term use of up to three days for a patient experiencing insomnia and anxiety at a dose of 1–2 mg at bedtime only; if that patient takes double the intended dose to induce sleep knowingly, this action constitutes misuse with respect to inappropriate use of lorazepam.

Prescription drug disorder is a medical condition that occurs when ongoing prescription misuse leads to clinical and functional impairment in either a temporary or permanent capacity depending on the prognosis of the condition, and often occurs before dependence (Schepis et al., 2020).

Physical dependence on a prescription drug occurs because the body adapts to regular exposure resulting in withdrawal symptoms when the drug is discontinued (Schepis et al., 2020).

Epidemiology

Over 54 million people have used prescription drugs at least once in their lifetime for nonmedical reasons, and over 50% of medications prescribed for patients are either taken incorrectly or not taken at all (Chibi et al., 2019). Similar to other parts of the world, prescription drug misuse is increasingly reported in sub-Saharan Africa. Although available data from sub-Saharan Africa is limited because of the lack of monitoring systems, evidence emerging from countries with available population surveys and treatment data shows a growing trend of PDM, including a possible switch from illicit drug use to PDM (2010a; UNODC, 2020). While synthetic opioids remain a problem in high-income countries, tramadol, an opioid analgesic, has increasingly been reported in illegal African and Asian markets; 87% of total global illegal pharmaceutical opioid seizures in 2016 were in Africa (UNODC, 2018).

PDM is associated with a range of adverse health outcomes, including infectious disease transmission, substance use disorders, mental disorders, and overdose deaths (UNODC, 2020). This problem is particularly concerning among adolescents and youths, and emerging evidence shows early misuse of prescription drugs is associated with substance dependence in adulthood (Perlmutter et al., 2018). For example, a cross-sectional study among young people in Ghana found that more than half of the respondents had used tramadol for nonmedical purposes and one-third of these users reported misusing nine to ten doses of tramadol per day (Elliason et al., 2018).

Comorbid mental health disorders are common among people with substance use disorder. The burden of mental disorders and substance use disorders in Africa was estimated at 19% of the total health burden and was the leading cause of years lived with disability in 2010 (Charlson et al., 2014). Although it is common for mental disorders to be associated with substance use and misuse, little is known about the onset of comorbid mental health conditions; therefore, causality cannot be determined.

Globally, overall drug use remains low among women compared to men. However, women are more likely to misuse prescription opioids and benzodiazepines than men (Degenhardt et al., 2019; UNODC, 2015). A systematic review of opioid use in Africa noted that most of the reviewed papers used predominantly male samples (Kurth et al., 2018). The scarcity of data on women with drug use disorders implies that women face barriers to accessing services, including methadone treatment. Therefore, there is a need for gender-sensitive research and policies exploring the specific needs of women.

Major advances in the management of HIV has evolved the disease into a chronic manageable disease, and people living with HIV (PLWH) are now living longer. However, chronic pain affects nearly 80% of PLWH, with the aetiology of pain attributed to multiple causes including HIV neuropathies, ARV side effects and HIV-associated disorders (Petit et al., 2018). Chronic pain among PLWH has been associated with functional disability, reduced quality of life, high health resource use, poor retention in care, and risk behaviours that can transmit HIV to others (Robinson-Papp et al., 2019). Although the presence of illicit drug use has been identified as a risk factor for opioid misuse in high-income countries, evidence from sub-Saharan Africa remains scarce. Given the high burden of HIV in sub-Saharan Africa, understanding PDM is necessary to improve health outcomes among PLWH.

Chronic pain is a common comorbidity among PLWH and has been implicated in PDM (Cunningham, 2018). Pain is experienced throughout the HIV disease trajectory, and opioids are commonly prescribed to PLWH at higher doses than are available to the general public (Edelman et al., 2013). A cross-sectional study conducted among PLWH in South Africa reported a high prevalence of drug diversion, with 23% of participants reporting PDM in the last 90 days (Chibi et al., 2020). Furthermore, a survey in 12 African countries showed clinicians were inadequately trained to prescribe pain medications for PLWH, which led to self-medication and drug misuse (Harding et al., 2010). Given that PLWH commonly experience chronic pain that necessitates long-term opioid prescription, opioid expansion needs to balance access, clinicians' skills, and regulation of opioids.

However, the authors for this chapter have identified in their practice that people on prescribed opioids, with multiple previous traumatic events, due to accidents, injury, and/or cancerous mutations, are more prone to opioid misuse. Recurrent use of opioids tends to cause dependence because there is an indistinct difference between misuse and effective chronic pain management. Additionally, PLWH tend to be associated with misuse of Efavirenz (an antiretroviral active medicine that is a characteristic ingredient for whoonga). An example to explain the aforementioned whoonga concept has been given in Chap. 7 under the subheading 'Smoking Whoonga, Wunga or Nyaope' and **Case Study 7.4: Whoonga, the Cruellest Drug of South African Slums.** Refer to Case Study 7.4 and answer the following question:

Stop and Reflect

1. From the case study blog, explain the key characteristics differentiating PDM, substance use, and dependence.

Major Classes of Misused Prescription Drugs

The commonly used drugs are divided into categories based on their pharmacological activity. Many prescription drugs can potentially be misused, including laxatives, steroids, antidepressants, and anticholinergics. However, this chapter focuses on commonly prescribed psychotropic drugs: prescription analgesics (opioids), stimulants (amphetamines), and sedatives-hypnotics (benzodiazepines and quaaludes).

Opioids

Opioids are commonly used as analgesic drugs to treat both acute and chronic pain. Opiates are alkaloids extracted from the poppy plant, and opioids comprise synthetic and semisynthetic compounds that work by binding to the *mu* receptor in cells producing effects such as analgesia (Sun et al., 2017). Although this class of medications is highly effective for managing severe pain, they are known to induce respiratory depression even when used therapeutically, and repeated exposure can lead to dependence (Sun et al., 2017).

The potential for misuse of opioid pain medications has complicated the prescription of opioids in the treatment of chronic pain and cancer. Misuse of opioids is a global public health issue. Opioid consumption is disproportionally high in high-income countries, with low-income countries consuming only 6% of the available global opioids (Manjiani et al., 2014). According to the UNODC (2018), 83% of the world has no access to opioid treatment for pain. Campaigns creating awareness for treating pain as the fifth vital sign increased opioid consumption for the treatment of pain in North America and Europe but the medical use of opioids remains stagnant in Africa (Kurth et al., 2018). However, multiple sub-Saharan African countries are reporting growing numbers of prescription opioid use disorders with opioid dependence as a major contributor to premature morbidity and mortality in sub-Saharan Africa (Degenhardt et al., 2014). Sharing contaminated drug injection equipment also increases the risk of contracting infectious diseases such as HIV/AIDS and hepatitis.

Accurate statistics for commonly misused prescription opioids in Africa remain scarce, but emerging evidence shows tramadol and codeine are increasingly trafficked and consumed in Africa. Several African countries, including Benin, Nigeria, Ghana, Togo, Sierra Leone, Cameroon, and the Ivory Coast (see Fig. 9.1) have been cited as countries with high demand for tramadol (Salm-Reifferscheidt, 2018). For example, in Nigeria, tramadol misuse has been reported at 54.4%, with the drug mostly sourced without prescription (Ibrahim et al., 2017). Tramadol use can produce both psychiatric and physical opioid-like effects. For decades, tramadol was considered to have low potential for dependence. However, tramadol dependence has been shown to occur after prolonged use and when used in large doses (WHO, 2014). In many African countries, tramadol is available over the counter (OTC) or via the internet without a prescription.

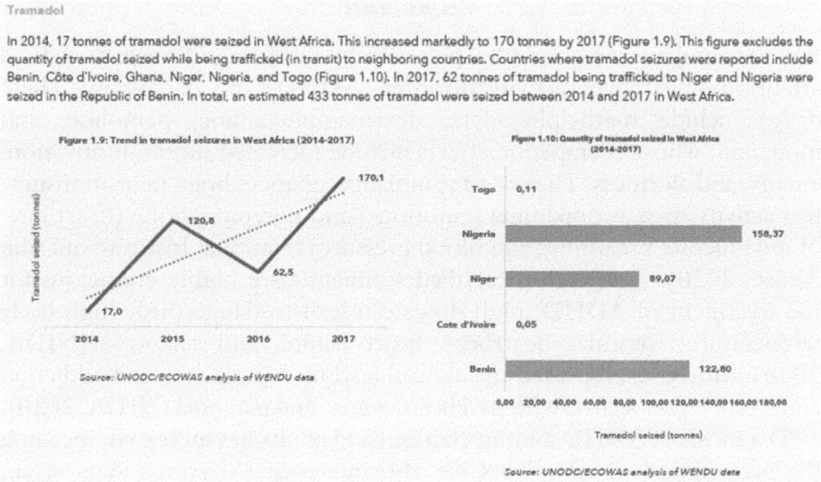
Tramadol

In 2014, 17 tonnes of tramadol were seized in West Africa. This increased markedly to 170 tonnes by 2017 (Figure 1.9). This figure excludes the quantity of tramadol seized while being trafficked (in transit) to neighboring countries. Countries where tramadol seizures were reported include Benin, Côte d'Ivoire, Ghana, Niger, Nigeria, and Togo (Figure 1.10). In 2017, 62 tonnes of tramadol being trafficked to Niger and Nigeria were seized in the Republic of Benin. In total, an estimated 433 tonnes of tramadol were seized between 2014 and 2017 in West Africa.

Fig. 9.1 Tramadol quantities seized in West Africa (UNODC, 2019)

Case Study 9.1: Tramadol Use in Ghana
In Ghana, tramadol misuse has been associated with a confluence of factors. As with other studies in the region, participants in that study cited peer pressure and curiosity as the main initiation drivers. Other motivations for tramadol misuse were perceived enhancement of sexual intercourse by treating premature ejaculation and ejaculation-related distress. Participants also admitted to using the drug for its euphoric effects, alertness, and treating low mood and fatigue. Furthermore, tramadol is affordable and readily available without a prescription.

Adapted from Peprah et al. (2020).

Stop and Reflect

1. How can governments control the illegal use of tramadol in their respective countries?
2. Would you use tramadol illegally given its pros and cons? Discuss.

Stimulants

Psychostimulants are typically prescribed in treating disorders such as attention-deficit hyperactivity disorder (ADHD) and narcolepsy. These drugs include methylphenidate, dextroamphetamine, pemoline, and modafinil, whose therapeutic effects include increased mood, motivation, energy, and alertness. The use of stimulants enhances brain neurotransmitters activity such as dopamine (emotions) and norepinephrine (heart rate, blood glucose, breathing, and blood pressure) (National Institute of Drug Abuse, 2020). Although prescribed stimulants are highly efficacious for the treatment of ADHD, high doses can lead to dangerously high body temperature, irregular heartbeat, heart failure, and seizures ((NIDA, 2020). Moreover, repeated misuse can lead to dependency and addiction and has been associated with psychosis, anger, and paranoia (NIDA, 2020).

Diagnosis of ADHD among children and adults has increased, meaning the prescription of stimulants has also increased (Martinez-Raga et al., 2017). However, misuse of prescription stimulants with amphetamine-like properties has been reported, particularly among adolescents and college students who misuse the drug in academic environments to improve concentration as well as recreationally for its euphoric and weight loss effects (Martinez-Raga et al., 2017). A study among undergraduate medical students in South Africa reported stimulant misuse (Retief & Verster, 2016). Furthermore, most participants in that study (Retief & Verster, 2016) who misused stimulants obtained the drugs from friends or classmates, although some reported other sources including over the counter (OTC) from pharmacies and the internet.

Central Nervous Depressants

This class of medicine is generally divided into categories based on their purpose rather than their pharmacotherapeutic properties. These medications are used to treat anxiety, panic attacks, stress reactions, and insomnia. Sedatives-hypnotics mainly include barbiturates, quaaludes, and sleep medications (e.g., zolpidem). Quaaludes such as methaqualone are currently rarely prescribed because of their highly addictive nature, but illegal manufacturing continues for recreational use in countries like South Africa (UNODC, 2010b). Adverse effects of methaqualone dependence include ataxia (loss of control of body movements), mental impairment, confusion, and poor judgement. Tranquillizers include benzodiazepines, muscle relaxants, and anti-anxiety medications. These central nervous system depressants slow brain activity causing dizziness, slurred speech, lowered blood pressure, depressed breathing, and memory loss (NIDA, 2020). Signs and symptoms of benzodiazepine overdose include impaired consciousness and ataxia. Clinically, flumazenil (a benzodiazepine antagonist) can be administered under monitored circumstances at a health facility with both human and clinical resources to reduce morbidity. Although benzodiazepines are not known to directly cause overdoses, they have been linked to some overdoses and deaths when used in combination with other drugs such as alcohol and opioids (NIDA, 2020). Evidence shows concurrent use of benzodiazepines with opioids has increased in the last two decades and contributes to significant deaths (Sun et al., 2017).

Prevention and Harm Reduction

PDM is a public health issue in sub-Saharan Africa, highlighting the need for increased pharmacovigilance and regulation at both clinical practice and pharmacy levels. Global awareness of trafficking and PDM is increasing, and there are calls to implement evidence-based strategies to prevent and reduce harm from drug misuse. Strategies include ensuring dispensing, risk screening, management, monitoring, and surveillance of prescribed drugs. However, complex political, structural, and socioeconomic factors influence drug use and the corresponding responses in the region result in slow progress in adopting evidence-based strategies. A review of medicine regulatory systems in sub-Saharan Africa showed a general lack of quality-monitoring programmes and a lack of regulatory harmonisation across countries (WHO, 2010).

The role of harm reduction is to reduce the injury associated with PDM. This includes increasing access to overdose reversal drugs and providing people who inject drugs with access to clean syringes, testing, and treatment services for HIV and hepatitis infection. Implementing harm reduction measures has been slow in most sub-Saharan African countries because of volatile legislative environments and lack of political will (Adelekan, 1998). Although testing for hepatitis B and C is offered in some countries like Kenya and hepatitis C testing and diagnosis is affordable, the current estimated costs of treatment for chronic hepatitis C are prohibitive in sub-Saharan Africa (Abdool, 2016). Several countries have made naloxone available in their emergency rooms or operating theatres as a means of reversing an opiate overdose. In Kenya, Mauritius, and Tanzania, naloxone is available at opioids substitution clinics or adjoining health facilities and piloted by outreach workers at the street level in Kenya (Abdool, 2016).

Treatment for Prescription Drug Disorders

Treatment for prescription drug disorders is tailored to the type of drug used. The development of a treatment plan for prescription drug disorders is based on assessing clinical history, a physical examination, and comorbid conditions. The treatment for the prescription opioid disorder is the same as that for a person with heroin use disorder. Opioid agonist medication (methadone) and opioid partial agonist (buprenorphine) are effective in treating opioid use disorders. There are no medications currently approved to treat stimulant or sedative use disorders, but behavioural therapies have shown promising results.

Case Study 9.2: Treating Codeine Misuse and Dependence in South Africa

There is a gap in the training of providers to treat codeine misuse disorder in South Africa. Results have shown that providers treated an average of 41 patients with codeine use disorder per year. Treatment modalities included detoxification, pharmacotherapy, cognitive behavioral therapy (CBT), interviewing, and psychodynamic therapy. CBT was the most common treatment offered. However, only 2 out of 20 providers had received training on how to treat codeine dependence. All participants admitted they would benefit from additional training on codeine misuse and dependence.

Adapted from Parry et al. (2017).

Stop and Reflect

1. What treatment modalities for PDM and dependence are available in your area?
2. What type of PDM training is needed for:
    (a) Doctors,
    (b) Nurses,
    (c) Pharmacists,
    (d) Mental health counsellors, and
    (e) Providers?

Justify your answers.

Case Study 9.3: Chronic Opioid Use after Surgery

Mr X is a 45-year-old man who was involved in a car accident with his wife and their 5-year-old son during the Easter holidays in 2008. His wife was deceased at the scene of the accident and their son survived with minor injuries. He presented to the local government hospital emergency room with complex open tibia fracture, extensive tissue loss, and arterial damage. He was rushed into surgery where he underwent a below knee amputation (BKA) operation.

(*continued*)

Case Study 9.3: (continued)

The timely BKA was successful in saving his life. Post-operation, Mr. X was prescribed morphine to manage pain and fluoxetine following trauma.

In 2010, Mr X went to a private hospital for assistance with severe phantom limb pain, lack of sleep, depressive episodes, suicidal ideation, and craving; he explained that only morphine helped. The prescriber added zolpidem as a sedative and hypnotic anti-depressant. To avoid being questioned, Mr X collects pain medication from a government facility and antidepressants from a private facility.

(R.W. Kimani, personal communication, August 20, 2020).

Stop and Reflect

1. How can we manage Mr. X's case effectively considering the disintegration between government and private facilities in sub-Saharan Africa?
2. Considering Mr. X is showing signs of PDM, what control measures can be implemented by:
   (a) Doctors,
   (b) Pharmacists,
   (c) Psychiatrists,
   (d) Psychologists,
   (e) Counsellors,
   (f) Government programmes/campaigns, and
   (g) Community?

   Justify your answers.

Summary

PDM is an increasing public health problem in sub-Saharan Africa. The sources of misused medications include informal networks, probably because of drug trafficking, dysregulation of drugs, and lack of clear prescription drug control policies. Adolescents, women, and those living with

HIV are at an increased risk for PDM. There is a gap in the availability of PDM disorders treatment and training of addiction providers in sub-Saharan Africa.

End of Chapter Questions

1. What are the likely sources of PDM medications in sub-Saharan Africa?
2. According to epidemiological reports from Africa, which opioids are most likely to be misused?
3. List some professional bodies in your country that can form an interdisciplinary team to aid in addressing PDM and dependence?
4. Do the countries in sub-Saharan Africa have appropriate human resources and infrastructure to manage misuse of drugs?
5. What are the differences between PDM and dependence? What are three ways that medicines can be misused? Provide examples.
6. What are the major pharmacological classes of drugs associated with PDM and how can they be managed to control emergency cases of abuse?
7. Briefly describe the impact of PDM based on its epidemiology in sub-Saharan Africa.
8. Explain the key characteristics differentiating PDM, substance use, and dependence.
9. How can we prevent PDM among:

    (a) Teens,
    (b) Young adults, and
    (c) Older adults?

References

Abdool, R. (2016). Policy change towards implementing harm reduction in sub-Saharan Africa. *International Journal of Drug Policy, 30*, 140–142.

Adelekan, M. L. (1998). Substance use, HIV infection and the harm reduction approach in sub-Saharan Africa. *International Journal of Drug Policy, 9*(5), 315–323. https://doi.org/10.1016/S0955-3959(98)00042-5.

Charlson, F. J., Diminic, S., Lund, C., Degenhardt, L., & Whiteford, H. A. (2014). Mental and substance use disorders in sub-Saharan Africa: Predictions of epidemiological changes and mental health workforce requirements for the next 40 years. *PLoS One, 9*(10), e110208.

Chibi, B., Torres, N., Sokhela, Z., & Mashamba-Thompson, T. (2019). Prescription drug diversion among people living with HIV: A systematic scoping review. *Public Health, 177*, 26–43.

Chibi, B., Yende-Zuma, N., & Mashamba-Thompson, T. P. (2020). Prevalence and correlates of prescription drug diversion and misuse among people living with HIV in the eThekwini district, KwaZulu-Natal, South Africa. *PLoS One, 15*(12), e0243718. https://doi.org/10.1371/journal.pone.0243718.

Compton, W. M., & Volkow, N. D. (2006). Abuse of prescription drugs and the risk of addiction. *Drug and Alcohol Dependence, 83*, S4–S7.

Cunningham, C. O. (2018). Opioids and HIV infection: From pain management to addiction treatment. *Topics in Antiviral Medicine, 25*(4), 143–146.

Degenhardt, L., Bharat, C., Glantz, M. D., Sampson, N. A., Scott, K., Lim, C. C., … Andrade, L. H. (2019). The epidemiology of drug use disorders cross-nationally: Findings from the WHO's World Mental Health Surveys. *International Journal of Drug Policy, 71*, 103–112.

Degenhardt, L., Charlson, F., Mathers, B., Hall, W. D., Flaxman, A. D., Johns, N., & Vos, T. (2014). The global epidemiology and burden of opioid dependence: Results from the global burden of disease 2010 study. *Addiction, 109*(8), 1320–1333. https://doi.org/10.1111/add.12551

Edelman, E. J., Gordon, K., Becker, W. C., Goulet, J. L., Skanderson, M., Gaither, J. R., … Fiellin, D. A. (2013). Receipt of opioid analgesics by HIV-infected and uninfected patients. *Journal of General Internal Medicine, 28*(1), 82–90. https://doi.org/10.1007/s11606-012-2189-z

Elliason, E., Sandow, B., Asechaab, T., Kpangkpari, S., & Asiaktiwen, R. (2018). Abuse and misuse of tramadol among the youth in the Wassa Amenfi west municipality in the Western region of Ghana. *International Journal of Psychological Research, 3*(7), 000181.

Harding, R., Powell, R. A., Kiyange, F., Downing, J., & Mwangi-Powell, F. (2010). Provision of pain- and symptom-relieving drugs for HIV/AIDS in sub-Saharan Africa. *Journal of Pain and Symptom Management, 40*(3), 405–415. https://doi.org/10.1016/j.jpainsymman.2009.12.025

Ibrahim, A., Yerima, M., Pindar, S., Onyencho, V., Ahmed, H., Machina, B., … Wakil, M. (2017). Tramadol abuse among patients attending an addiction clinic in North-Eastern Nigeria: Outcome of a four year retrospective study. *Advances in Psychology and Neuroscience, 2*(1-2), 31–37.

Kurth, A. E., Cherutich, P., Conover, R., Chhun, N., Bruce, R. D., & Lambdin, B. H. (2018). The opioid epidemic in Africa and its impact. *Current Addiction Reports, 5*(4), 428–453. https://doi.org/10.1007/s40429-018-0232-9.

Manjiani, D., Paul, D. B., Kunnumpurath, S., Kaye, A. D., & Vadivelu, N. (2014). Availability and utilization of opioids for pain management: Global issues. *The Ochsner Journal, 14*(2), 208–215.

Martinez-Raga, J., Ferreros, A., Knecht, C., de Alvaro, R., & Carabal, E. (2017). Attention-deficit hyperactivity disorder medication use: Factors involved in prescribing, safety aspects and outcomes. *Therapeutic Advances in Drug Safety, 8*(3), 87–99. https://doi.org/10.1177/2042098616679636

National Institute of Drug Abuse. (2020, June 25). *The science of drug use and addiction: The basics.* https://www.drugabuse.gov/publications/media-guide/science-drug-use-addiction-basics

Parry, C. D., Rich, E., Van Hout, M. C., & Deluca, P. (2017). Codeine misuse and dependence in South Africa: Perspectives of addiction treatment providers. *South African Medical Journal, 107*(5), 451–456.

Peprah, P., Agyemang-Duah, W., Appiah-Brempong, E., Akwasi, A. G., & Morgan, A. K. (2020). "With tramadol, i ride like a jaguar": A qualitative study of motivations for nonmedical purpose tramadol use among commercial vehicle operators in Kumasi, Ghana. *Substance Abuse Treatment, Prevention, and Policy, 15*(1), 49. https://doi.org/10.1186/s13011-020-00292-4

Perlmutter, A. S., Bauman, M., Mantha, S., Segura, L. E., Ghandour, L., & Martins, S. S. (2018). Nonmedical prescription drug use among adolescents: Global epidemiological evidence for prevention, assessment, diagnosis, and treatment. *Current Addiction Reports, 5*(2), 120–127. https://doi.org/10.1007/s40429-018-0194-y

Petit, N., Enel, P., Ravaux, I., Darque, A., Baumstarck, K., Bregigeon, S., & Retornaz, F. (2018). Frail and pre-frail phenotype is associated with pain in older HIV-infected patients. *Medicine, 97*(6), e9852.

Peyraud, N., Rafael, F., Parker, L. A., Quere, M., Alcoba, G., Korff, C., … Serafini, M. (2017). An epidemic of dystonic reactions in Central Africa. *The Lancet Global Health, 5*(2), e137–e138.

Retief, M., & Verster, C. (2016). Prevalence and correlates of nonmedical stimulants and related drug use in a sample of south African undergraduate medical students. *The South African Journal of Psychiatry, 22*(1), 795–795. https://doi.org/10.4102/sajpsychiatry.v22i1.795

Robinson-Papp, J., Aberg, J., Benn, E. K. T., Bryan, A., Cedillo, G., Chikamoto, Y., … Fisher, J. (2019). Decreasing risk among HIV patients on opioid therapy for chronic pain: Development of the TOWER intervention for HIV care providers. *Contemporary Clinical Trials Communications, 16*, 100468. https://doi.org/10.1016/j.conctc.2019.100468.

Salm-Reifferscheidt, L. (2018). Tramadol: Africa's opioid crisis. *The Lancet, 391*(10134), 1982–1983. https://doi.org/10.1016/S0140-6736(18)31073-0.

Schepis, T. S., Klare, D. L., Ford, J. A., & McCabe, S. E. (2020). Prescription drug misuse: Taking a lifespan perspective. *Substance Abuse: Research and Treatment, 14*, 1–28.

Sun, E. C., Dixit, A., Humphreys, K., Darnall, B. D., Baker, L. C., & Mackey, S. (2017). Association between concurrent use of prescription opioids and benzodiazepines and overdose: Retrospective analysis. *BMJ, 356*, j760.

United Nation Office on Drugs and Crime. (2015). *Status and trend analysis of illicit drug markets.* https://www.unodc.org/documents/wdr2015/WDR15_Drug_use_health_consequences.pdf
United Nation Office on Drugs and Crime. (2019). *West African epidemiology network on drug use (WENDU) report: Statistics and trends on illicit drug use and supply 2014-2017.* https://www.unodc.org/documents/westandcentralafrica//WENDU_REPORT_VF_V5_291019_FINAL_VERSION.pdf
United Nations Office of Drug and Crime. (2018). *World drug report 2018: Opioid crisis, prescription drug abuse expands; cocaine and opium hit record highs.* https://www.unodc.org/unodc/en/press/releases/2018/June/world-drug-report-2018_-opioid-crisis%2D%2Dprescription-drug-abuse-expands-cocaine-and-opium-hit-record-highs.html
United Nations Office of Drugs and Crime. (2010a). *The nonmedical use of prescription drugs: Policy direction issues.* https://www.unodc.org/docs/treatment/Prescription_Drugs_background_paper.pdf
United Nations Office of Drugs and Crime. (2010b). *Recommended methods for the identification and analysis of methaqualone/mecloqualone.* https://www.unodc.org/documents/scientific/Methaqualone_ST_NAR_15_Rev1.pdf
United Nations Office of Drugs and Crime. (2020). World drug report 2020. https://wdr.unodc.org/wdr2020/field/WDR20_Booklet_2.pdf
World Health Organization. (2010). *Regulating harmonization; updating medicines regulatory systems in sub-Saharan African countries.* https://www.who.int/medicines/technical_briefing/tbs/regulatory_harmonization_DrugInfo2010_Vol24_1.pdf?ua=1
World Health Organization. (2014). *Tramadol: Update review report.* Paper presented at the Expert Committee on Drug Dependence Thirty-sixth Meeting Geneva.

CHAPTER 10

Prevention of Substance Use among the Youth: A Public Health Priority

Kegomoditswe Manyanda, David Sidney Mangwegape, Wazha Dambe, and Ketwesepe Hendrick

Abstract Excessive substance consumption is a growing public health concern globally as it alters the optimal function of the human brain, leading to severe physiological, psychological, and social problems. Compelling evidence shows that certain groups of people may be more vulnerable to substance use and misuse than members of the general population. These groups, sometimes referred to as "special populations" have unique health concerns that require exceptional attention in the prevention of substance use/misuse. Special populations include among others the poor or

K. Manyanda (✉)
Aspire Health Services Group, Gaborone, Botswana

D. S. Mangwegape
Institute of Health Sciences-Lobatse, Department of Psychiatric Mental Health Nursing, Lobatse, Botswana

W. Dambe
BOSASNet, Gaborone, Botswana

K. Hendrick
Department of Psychology, University of Botswana, Gaborone, Botswana

M. Mhaka-Mutepfa (ed.), *Substance Use and Misuse in sub-Saharan Africa*, https://doi.org/10.1007/978-3-030-85732-5_10

homeless, women, young adults or teenagers, the elderly, and trauma survivors. The focus of this chapter is on the prevention of substance use and misuse in young people and teenagers, including those that are homeless. Young people engage in substance use due to peer pressure or as a way of experimentation and, therefore, are more vulnerable. Several factors linked to substance use disorders among teenagers are also discussed. The chapter also utilises both primary and secondary data focusing on substance-related disorders in adolescents, enhancing resilience and methods for reducing risk behaviour. Challenges as well as best practices and recommendations for addressing stigma, treatment needs, the support structures needed for effective prevention of substance use in young people are also discussed.

Keywords Substance use disorders • Prevention • Intervention • Special populations • Health • Evidence-based treatment • Management • Young people

Introduction

Substance use is a significant public health concern and in both developed and developing countries. The Executive Director of United Nations Office on Drugs and Crime (UNODC) highlighted that vulnerable and marginalised groups (e.g., the youth, women, older people, and the poor) bear the brunt of a much larger problem (O'Dowd, 2020). The United Nations defines "youth" as persons aged 15–24 years, with the definition varying in different countries worldwide (United Nations, 2008). According to the World Drug Report, 269 million people used drugs worldwide in 2018 (UNODC, 2020). The report further highlighted that adolescents and young adults were the most vulnerable to substance use and experienced devastating consequences on account of their developing brains. Cannabis was estimated to be used by 192 million people in 2018 (Riva et al., 2018; UNODC, 2020). The overwhelming number of those affected was the youth.

The problem of substance use has been a concern among youth in sub-Saharan Africa (Ludick & Amone-P'Olak, 2016). As observed by Keetile (2020), the common health risk behaviour among adolescents is substance use, particularly alcohol. The youth are prominently affected and have the highest prevalence (Selemogwe et al., 2014). A global review by UNODC and systematic reviews in Africa revealed that the age of debut for substance use is 15–18 years (Olashore et al., 2018; UNODC, 2020). Earlier studies in African countries such as Nigeria showed that youths started using substances from the ages of 12–24 years (Babalola et al., 2013). Riva et al. (2018) posited that illicit drug use has been documented as a problem in sub-Saharan Africa as it also results in adverse consequences, especially if there is early onset.

Impact of Early Onset of Substance Use

Early onset of substance use such as alcohol has been linked to both physical and mental health-related challenges (Swahn et al., 2013). Individuals with substance use disorders (SUDs) may intensively utilise criminal justice system resources as well as other public services and programmes including public mental health and general medical care services (Slade et al., 2008), thereby resulting in high health costs. In addition, the treatment of SUD among young people may extend across multiple agencies within the public sector, increasing health costs further.

The age of onset is also related to consequences experienced in later life (Slade et al., 2008). The authors posited that age of onset for use of alcohol and illicit drugs can be valuable in identifying individuals at risk of severe substance use/misuse in adulthood. This means that it is possible to pre-empt an individual's gradual level of substance use based on when they started using. Understanding the factors contributing to substance use is vital in developing mitigation strategies. The contributing factors range from biological, social, and psychological influences.

Risk and Protective Factors Associated with Substance Use in Young People

Risk factors for the onset of substance use among young people include peer pressure, exposure to substances, genetic predisposition, and adverse early life experiences (Swadi, 1999). The homeless and street children endure difficult circumstances leaving their home on account of abuse and poverty which make them more vulnerable to substance use (Cumber & Tsoka-Gwegweni, 2015; Hodgson et al., 2013). Protective factors, in contrast, help in averting the use of substances. Previous researchers in Botswana (Riva et al., 2018) and a meta-analysis of global studies (Valero de Vicente et al., 2017) found that support from friends, family and school attachment, and optimism about the future was associated with delayed substance use/misuse. The positive traits by parents can be emulated and thus a child will be able to communicate effectively and make good choices.

Case Study 10.1: Street Children and Substance Use
PP is an 18-year-old male who left his home when he was only 14 years old. He lost both his parents in a car accident at 6 years and was raised by his uncle. He was neglected and abused unlike the other children at home. He eventually left home and stayed on the streets. He sniffed glue and occasionally had a puff of dagga from his streets mates. He was brought to the emergency ward smelling terribly after suffering from hypothermia. His mates thought he had contracted COVID-19. However, PP hand taken hand **sanitizer** used for preventing the spread of COVID-19 that he stole from a supermarket so that he would get drunk. He was also vomiting, coughing, and had stomach aches. He was treated for methanol toxicity.

(K. Manyanda, personal communication, July 17, 2020).

Stop and Reflect

1. Discuss PP's risk factors and protective factors.
2. Discuss issues that affect street children and how they rely on drugs.
3. How would you assist PP to get off the streets and live a normal life?
4. What should governments and civil societies do to help street children?
5. How would you educate your peers on the effects of hand sanitizer when ingested?

The problem of street kids is a universal problem in sub-Saharan Africa. According to Souza et al. (2010), there is dearth of evidence of programmes targeting street youth because it is cumbersome to describe the feasibility and outcome of services rendered to youth in most low- to middle-income countries, let alone those that live on the streets. Children living on the streets might be unaware of the harmful effects of ingesting substances, particularly hand sanitizers, therefore the need for educating the youths.

Strategies to Prevent Substance Use in Youths

Prevention of substance use among young people is broadly set to ensure that they realise their potential in life and make full use of their talents (UNODC, 2013). Evidence-based strategies often have multiple outcomes; delayed initiation of substance use amongst them. These strategies are entrenched on a framework based on the social-ecological approach adapted from Bronfenbrenner's ecological systems theory (see UNODC, 2017). The theory states that a child's development is affected by their interactions with their microsystem (immediate environment such as family and school), mesosystem (connections between structures in microsystem), exosystem (larger, indirect environment), macrosystem (social and cultural values), and chronosystem (changes with time and age) (Bronfenbrenner, 1992). Therefore, substance use prevention programmes should incorporate the youths' internal state, family, school, larger systems such as community organisations, cultural beliefs and social norms concerning substance use across childhood and early adulthood developmental stages. Table 10.1 summarises evidence-based strategies for prevention of substance use incorporating the microsystem, mesosystem, macrosystem, exosystem, and chronosystem levels.

Table 10.1 further shows that substance use prevention strategies are imperative from the prenatal stage through to adulthood and from the family level to the health sector level, suggesting that prevention is an ongoing process at all stages and levels of development. It further provides evidence that most substance use prevention strategies are focused on young people from middle childhood to adolescent years. UNODC (2019) suggests that prevention strategies based on scientific evidence working with families, schools, and communities can ensure that children and youth, especially the most marginalised and poor, grow healthy and safe into adulthood and old age. UNODC (2019) posited that for every dollar spent on prevention; at least ten dollars can be saved in future health expenses.

From anecdotal experience, there have not been many evidence-based substance use prevention strategies in most African countries. Many of the activities in most countries included general education of adolescents on use of substances by professionals, guidance and counselling teachers, police officers and individuals who have used substances before. This has been criticised by the UNODC (2013), which asserts that substance use prevention is complex because education as a stand-alone activity has not

Table 10.1 Summary of Evidence-Based Strategies Identified in the UNODC/WHO International Standards on Drug Use Prevention

<table>
<tr><th></th><th>Prenatal & infancy</th><th>Early childhood</th><th>Middle childhood</th><th>Early adolescence</th><th>Adolescence</th><th>Adulthood</th></tr>
<tr><td>Family</td><td>Prenatal & infancy visitation</td><td></td><td colspan="2">Parenting skills</td><td></td><td></td></tr>
<tr><td></td><td>Interventions for pregnant women</td><td></td><td></td><td></td><td></td><td></td></tr>
<tr><td>School</td><td></td><td>Early childhood education</td><td>Personal & social skills education</td><td colspan="2">Prevention education based on social competence and influence</td><td></td></tr>
<tr><td></td><td></td><td></td><td>Classroom management</td><td></td><td>Addressing individual vulnerabilities</td><td></td></tr>
<tr><td></td><td></td><td></td><td>Policies to keep children in school</td><td colspan="2">School-wide programmes to enhance school attachment</td><td></td></tr>
<tr><td></td><td></td><td></td><td></td><td colspan="3">School policies on substance use</td></tr>
<tr><td>Community</td><td></td><td></td><td></td><td colspan="3">Alcohol & tobacco policies</td></tr>
<tr><td></td><td colspan="6">Community-based multi-component initiatives</td></tr>
<tr><td></td><td></td><td></td><td></td><td colspan="3">Media campaigns</td></tr>
<tr><td></td><td></td><td></td><td></td><td colspan="2">Mentoring</td><td></td></tr>
<tr><td></td><td></td><td></td><td></td><td></td><td colspan="2">Prevention programmes in entertainment venues</td></tr>
<tr><td>Workplace</td><td></td><td></td><td></td><td></td><td colspan="2">Workplace prevention programmes</td></tr>
<tr><td>Health sector</td><td>Interventions for pregnant women</td><td></td><td colspan="2">Addressing mental health disorders</td><td></td><td></td></tr>
<tr><td></td><td></td><td></td><td></td><td colspan="3">Brief intervention</td></tr>
</table>

Adapted from UNODC (2019)

been effective. In South Africa, strides have been made in addressing the problem where several interventions including provision of safe shelter and proper nutrition help to prevent substance use among street children and youths have been implemented (Cumber & Tsoka-Gwegweni, 2015). Mufune (2002) suggested a multi-sectored and integrated approach.

An Integrated Approach to Substance Use Prevention

An integrated approach as suggested by Mufune (2002) could be developed through a step-by-step process. Such a process should comprise needs assessment, organising, planning, implementation, and evaluation phases (Olawole-Isaac et al., 2018).

The Needs Assessment Phase: A thorough investigation into the risk factors predisposing youth of different communities to substance use is a vital step in putting together a holistic approach to substance use prevention (Olawole-Isaac et al., 2018). Exploration of protective factors, availability of resources as well as gaps in already established programmes is another important aspect to consider (UNODC, 2017). Additionally, the readiness of the communities, the openness they have to the interventions as they are a central part of the intervention, as well the policies surrounding substance use (UNODC, 2017) should be considered. The information from the assessments will determine the type of help required, enable measuring community readiness, and devise appropriate intervention. This includes gathering stakeholders (e.g., community leaders, teachers, parents) and holding meetings, taking surveys, and sharing benefits of the interventions.

The Organising Phase: This step entails sourcing support from stakeholders and the wider community to prepare for the planning phase (UNODC, 2017). In this phase, stakeholders such as private and government organisations are briefed on the idea in search of their support for the communities (UNODC, 2017). For example, in Botswana, organisations such as the Botswana Substance Abuse Support Network (BOSASNet) and the Anti-Tobacco Network (ATN) are key stakeholders in disseminating information about substances and the effects they have on the health of youth.

The Planning Phase: In this step, the main goal is to identify the vision of the prevention strategy and how the evaluation of the intervention will be undertaken (Olawole-Isaac et al., 2018). The data from the assessment phase is key as it will dictate which areas to start with, where resources are needed, time frames, and what needs to be done and how (UNODC, 2017).

The Implementation Phase: All the community members and relevant stakeholders come together to turn the plan into action especially at family and school level. Most of the young people spend a great deal of time at home and school; thus, school-based, and family-based prevention programmes are pertinent.

School-Based Substance Use Prevention Programmes: As observed by UNODC (2013), schools are an important target for prevention activities. There are diverging views on the availability of programmes dealing with substance use prevention in Africa. Gotsang et al. (2017) claim that most schools do not have strategies to deal with substances; a point refuted by

Diraditsile and Mabote (2017) who argue that there are school-based interventions, although they have not been effective in most countries. For instance, in some Low to Middle Income Countries (LMICs) (e.g., Zimbabwe and Botswana), there is peer approach to counselling for teens (Rose-Clarke et al., 2019). Existing trials have mixed results, with the most promising evidence supporting work with peer facilitators to improve adolescent mental health and reduce substance use and violence (Rose-Clarke et al., 2019). Despite the contradictions, there are several school-based programmes that can be used in substance use prevention which include Drug Abuse Resistance Education (DARE), Project Adolescent Learning Experiences Resistance Training, Life Skills Training (LST), the Alcohol Prevention Trial, and Project Choice (Tremblay et al., 2020). Evidence-based education is entrenched upon life skills and offers personal social skills, class management, resistance, and communication skills. Students should be taught skills which will help them resist peer pressure from pre-school years to early adulthood. During early adolescence, prevention education based on social competence and the enhancement of school attachment can be utilised.

Life Skills Training (LST) Programme: This programme entails teaching students general social and personal skills including drug resistance skills (Nsimba & Massele, 2012). It is basically a universal programme that addresses students at middle school or junior high levels and research on its effectiveness has been conducted (Griffin & Botvin, 2010). The LST programme is present in various sub-Saharan countries (e.g., South Africa, Tanzania, and Botswana) (WHO, 2003). In Botswana, the LST programme has been carried out through a partnership between the Centre for Disease Control (CDC) and the Ministry of Education and Skills Development (MOESD). Curricula for Standard 5 were developed and Life Skills were also developed for upper primary and secondary school students. The programmes empower young people and help in the pursuit of preventing substance use and misuse.

Family-Based Substance Use Prevention Programmes: Family skills training is often focused on the entire family and is targeted at enhancing positive family relationships, supervision, and communication within the family (UNODC, 2009) since family is a protective factor (Kumpfer, 2014).

Young people are impressionable; thus, family-based prevention programmes aim to solidify young people's resilience against peer pressure. These programmes have been found to be effective in helping young people shun substance use/misuse as well as adolescent delinquency (Kumpfer, 2014).

Antenatal, Infancy, and Middle Childhood Intervention: It is of utmost importance to pay particular attention to antenatal care and reduce substance use during pregnancy (Gilinsky et al., 2011). In most countries (e.g., Zimbabwe, Botswana, and South Africa), there are brief morning addresses by nurses in antenatal clinics where they include use/misuse of substances during pregnancy (personal communication). Additionally, parenting skills often take centre stage during middle childhood. Parents are mentored to monitor and supervise children's activities and to set age-appropriate limits on behaviour which goes a long way in preventing the onset of substance use (Lochman & van den Steenhoven, 2002).

The Evaluation Phase: Evaluation is done by looking at the initial goal of the intervention. In this case the goal is to reduce or delay early onset of substance use and minimise the occurrence of SUD (UNODC, 2017). Therefore, the evaluation phase will comprise conducting surveys to evaluate the impact of the intervention. Once again, the scientific method would be employed, using statistics of before and after the intervention, conducting qualitative assessments on the communities' experiences, and noting improvements as well as areas that still have gaps (Fry et al., 2018). In approaching substance use prevention in this integrated way, it can be expected that this intervention would be effective. However, it is also important that stigma against SUD be addressed as it has implications for the efficacy of substance use prevention and SUD treatment.

Stigma Against Substance Use Disorders

Stigma is broad and encompasses three main constructs; stereotypes, prejudice, and discrimination. Stigma has a huge influence in worsening or undermining population health outcomes and can be a major barrier to

Case Study 10.2: Living with Stigma
YB is a 20-year-old male recently diagnosed with dagga induced psychosis and has been undergoing counselling at the local psychiatric hospital. Ever since undergoing treatment, he has not been adequately involved in the family affairs and was at one point cast as crazy. He is not given money with family insinuating that he will buy dagga despite him needing money for pertinent issues. Last week he went to a clinic for his common cold symptoms and he overheard nurses saying that they will attend to him later as he is "just another dagga case"(*isidhakwa*)!

(D.S. Mangwegape, personal communication, March 15, 2021)

treatment access (Stangl et al., 2019). Language has also been seen to potentiate the gravity of stigma on substance use (Zwick et al., 2020). Words like *letagwa* and *letlhapelwa* (Setswana, Botswana), *chidhakwa and isidhakwa* (Shona and Ndebele, Zimbabwe), and *nsadweam* and *nnubɔnenomfoɔ* (Akan, Ghana) meaning addict or drunkard are deemed derogatory and stigmatising and should thus not be used to refer to individuals with SUD.

Stop and Reflect

1. There are high levels of stigma on people using alcohol, cannabis, methamphetamine, and heroin. Discuss how to eradicate stigma and help users stop the habit.
2. What are the societal expectations of users?
3. People who have SUD are said to have mental illness in most African countries. Distinguish between SUD and mental illness.

Addressing Stigma Against SUD

There are several frameworks that can be used to address stigma in substance use prevention. One such framework is the Health Stigma and Discrimination framework. As observed by Stangl et al. (2019), the framework is used widely and can respond effectively to addressing poor health outcomes caused by stigma. In comparison to other models, this framework seeks to refrain from making a distinction between those being stigmatised and those who stigmatise (Weiss as cited by Stangl et al., 2019). The framework highlights that the stigmatisation process constitutes domains that include drivers, facilitators, and manifestations (Stangl et al., 2019).

Drivers are the negative concepts about SUD. For example, an individual diagnosed with dagga-induced psychosis may feel that he is not productive because of his dependence. Facilitators often include issues surrounding health policies and cultural norms, among others. Substance use stigma may be borne from communities' view of dependence disorders not being illnesses, which creates prejudice against those who have been diagnosed with SUD. Manifestations will be the next domain characterised by stigma experiences and practices. Those diagnosed with SUD will experience stigma through self-stigma (own perceptions) and through others who may label them as addicts.

People diagnosed with SUD may not be given access to certain services because of dependence problems. They may be denied access to justice and quality healthcare. The stigma practices may then lead to unfair policies and legislation that disadvantage them. For instance, whipping of teens (those caught using substances, e.g., alcohol and cigarettes) in schools and customary courts without providing any other means of helping them to quit substances, may make them turn to substances again to deal with the physical pain and humiliation (L. Kenosi, personal communication, June 20, 2021). Therefore, stigma should be addressed holistically through, for instance, public education, avoiding labelling tendencies, advocating for non-discriminative laws and policies (Zwick et al., 2020), and continuous education among healthcare workers themselves.

Conclusion

This chapter extensively discussed the prevention of substance use and misuse in young people including street children. Young people have been seen to engage in substance use/misuse due to risk factors like peer pressure and genetic predisposition, among others. Protective factors that are mostly centred around parenting skills that cushion against the risk of SUD are discussed. Other strategies at family and school level that strive to enhance resilience among young people to reduce risky behaviour have also been explored. Dealing with stigma is also pivotal in ensuring effective treatment outcomes and access.

End of Chapter Questions

1. At what age/stage should substance use prevention be started?
2. What prevention strategies exist in your community?
3. Are there any programmes in place to address the phenomenon of street kids and their use of substances?
4. Discuss how you can mitigate stigma with regard to substance use/ misuse in your communities.

References

Babalola, E. O., Ogunwale, A., & Akinhami, A. (2013). Pattern of psychoactive substance use among university students in South-Western Nigeria. *Journal of Behavioural Health, 2*(4), 344–342. https://doi.org/10.5455/jbh.20130921013013.

Bronfenbrenner, U. (1992). Ecological systems theory. In R. Vasta (Ed.), *Six theories of child development: Revised formulations and current issues* (pp. 187–249). Jessica Kinsley Publishers.

Cumber, S. N., & Tsoka-Gwegweni, S. N. (2015). The health profile of street children in Africa: A literature review. *Journal of Public Health in Africa, 6*(2), 566. https://doi.org/10.4081.jphia.2015.566

Diraditsile, K., & Mabote, O. (2017). Alcohol and substance abuse in secondary schools in Botswana: The need for social workers in the school system. *Journal of Sociology, Psychology and Anthropology in Practice, 8*(2), 90–102.

Fry, C., Nikpay, S., Leslie, E., & Buntin, M. (2018). Evaluating community-based health improvement programs. *Health Affairs, 37*(1), 22–29.

Gilinsky, A., Swanson, V., & Power, K. (2011). Interventions delivered during antenatal care to reduce alcohol consumption during pregnancy: A systematic review. *Addiction Research & Theory, 19*(3), 235–250. https://doi.org/10.3109/16066359.2010.507894.

Gotsang, G., Mashalla, Y., & Seloilwe, E. (2017). Perceptions of school going adolescents about substance abuse in Ramotswa, Botswana. *Journal of Public Health and Epidemiology, 9*(6), 151–160. https://doi.org/10.5899/JPHE2017.0930

Griffin, K. W., & Botvin, G. J. (2010). Evidence based interventions for preventing substance use disorders in adolescents. *Child Adolescent Psychiatry Clinics of North America, 19*(5), 505–526. https://doi.org/10.1016/j.chc.2010.03.005

Hodgson, K. J., Shelton, K. H., Van den Bree, M. B., & Los, F. J. (2013). Psychopathology in young people experiencing homelessness: A systematic review. *American Journal of Public Health, 103*, e24–e37.

Keetile, M. (2020). Patterns and correlates of health risk behaviours among adolescents in Botswana: 2001–2013. *Vulnerable Children and Youth Studies*. https://doi.org/10.1080/17450128.2020.1752961

Kumpfer, K. L. (2014). Family based interventions for the prevention of substance abuse and other impulse control disorders in girls. *ISRN Addiction*. https://doi.org/10.1155/2014/308789

Lochman, J. E., & van den Steenhoven, A. (2002). Family-based approaches to substance abuse prevention. *The Journal of Primary Prevention, 23*, 49–114. https://doi.org/10.1023/A:1016591216363

Ludick, W. K., & Amone-P'Olak, K. (2016). Temperament and the risk of alcohol, tobacco and cannabis use among university students in Botswana. *African Journal of Drug & Alcohol Studies, 15*(1), 21–35.

Mufune, P. (2002). Street youth in Southern Africa. *International Social Science Journal*. https://doi.org/10.1111/1468-2451.002

Nsimba, S. E. D., & Massele, A. Y. (2012). A review on school-based interventions for alcohol, tobacco and other drugs (ATOD) in the United States of America; can developing countries in Africa adopt these preventive programs based on ATOD approaches? *Journal of Addiction Research and Therapy*. https://doi.org/10.4172/2155-6105.S2-007

O'Dowd, A. (2020). Drug misuse rose 30% in past decade and COVID-19 could worsen situation: UN report warns. *British Medical Journal*. https://doi.org/10.1136/bmj.m2631

Olashore, A. A., Ogunwobi, O., Totego, E., & Opondo, P. R. (2018). Psychoactive substance use among first-year students in a Botswana university: Pattern and correlates. *BMC Psychiatry, 18*, 270. https://doi.org/10.1186/s12888-018-1844-2

Olawole-Isaac, A., Ogundipe, O., Amoo, O., & Adeloye, D. (2018). Substance use among adolescents in sub-Saharan Africa: A systematic review and meta-analysis. *South African Journal of Child Health, 1*(12), 79–84. https://doi.org/10.7196/SAJCH.2018.v12i2.1524

Riva, K., Allen-Taylor, L., Schupmann, W. D., Mphele, S., Moshashane, N., & Lowenthal, E. D. (2018). Prevalence and predictors of alcohol and drug use among secondary school students in Botswana: A cross sectional study. *BMC Public Health, 18*, 1396. https://doi.org/10.1186/s12889-018-6263-2

Rose-Clarke, K., Bentley, A., Marston, C., & Prost, A. (2019). Peer-facilitated community-based interventions for adolescent health in low- and middle-income countries: A systematic review. *PLoS One, 14*(1), e0210468. https://doi.org/10.1371/journal.pone.0210468

Selemogwe, M., Mphele, S., & Manyanda, K. (2014). Drug use patterns and socio-demographic profits of substance users: Findings from a substance abuse treatment programme in Gaborone, Botswana. *African Journal of Drug & Alcohol Studies, 13*(1) 43–53.

Slade, E. P., Stuart, E. A., Salkever, D. S., Karakus, M., Green, K. M., & Ialongo, N. (2008). Impacts of age of onset of substance use disorders on risk of adult incarceration among disadvantaged urban youth: A propensity score matching approach. *Drugs and Alcohol Dependence, 95*(1–2), 1–13. https://doi.org/10.1016/j.drugalcdep.2007.11.019

Stangl, A. L., Eearnshaw, V. A., Logie, C. H., Van Brakel, W., Simbayi, L. C., Barre, I., & Dovidio, J. F. (2019). The health stigma and discrimination framework: A global, cross cutting framework to inform research, intervention development, and policy on health-related stigmas. *BMC Medicine, 17*(31). https://doi.org/10.1186/s129-019-1271-3

Souza, R., Porten, K., Nicholas, S. & Grais, R. (2010). Outcomes for street children and youth under multidisciplinary care in a drop in centre in Tegucigalpa, Honduras. *International Journal of Social Psychiatry*, 1–8. https://doi.org/10.1177/0020764010382367

Swadi, H. (1999). Individual risk factors for adolescent substance use. *Drug and Alcohol Dependence, 55*(3), 209–224. https://doi.org/10.1016/S0376-8716(99)00017-4

Swahn, M. H., Bossarte, R. M., Palmier, J. B., & Yao, H. (2013). Co-occurring physical fighting and suicide attempts among U.S. high school students: Examining patterns of early alcohol use initiation and current binge drinking. *The Western Journal of Emergency Medicine, 14*(4), 341–346. https://doi.org/10.5811/westjem.2013.3.15705

Tremblay, M., Baydala, L., Khan, M., Currie, C., Morley, K., Burkholder, C., … Stillar, A. (2020). Primary substance use prevention programs for children and youth: A systematic review. *Paediatrics, 146*(3). https://doi.org/10.1542/peds.2019-2747

United Nations. (2008). *Definition of youth.* United Nations. https://www.un.org/esa/socdev/documents/youth/fact-sheets/youth-definition.pdf

United Nations Office on Drugs and Crime. (2009). *Guide to implementing family skills training programmes for drug abuse prevention.* United Nations Office on Drugs and Crime. https://www.unodc.org/documents/prevention/family-guidelines-E.pdf

United Nations Office on Drugs and Crime. (2013). *International standards on drug use prevention.* United Nations Office on Drugs and Crime.

United Nations Office on Drugs and Crime. (2017). *Prevention of drug use and treatment of drug use disorders in rural settings: Revised version.* United Nations Office on Drugs and Crime.

United Nations Office on Drugs and Crime. (2019). *Summary table of evidence-based strategies identified in the UNODC/ WHO international standards on drug use prevention.* United Nations Office on Drugs and Crime.

United Nations Office on Drugs and Crime. (2020). *World drug report.* United Nations Office on Drugs and Crime. https://wdr2020.index.html

Valero de Vicente, M., Lluis, B. B., Orte Socias, M. D. M., & Amer Fernandez, J. A. (2017). Meta-analysis of family-based selective prevention programs for drug consumption in adolescence. *Psicothema, 29*(3), 299–305. https://doi.org/10.7334/psicothema2016.275

World Health Organisation. (2003). *Substance use in Southern Africa: Knowledge, attitudes, practices and opportunities for intervention.* World Health Organisation.

Zwick, J., Appleseth, H., & Arndt, S. (2020). Stigma: How it affects the substance use disorder patient. *Substance Abuse Treatment Prevention Policy, 15*, 50. https://doi.org/10.1186/s13011-020-00288-0

CHAPTER 11

Prevention and Intervention for Substance Use/Misuse

Katlego Lone Maikano, Refilwe Pearl Mogomotsi, Kabo Diraditsile, and Refilwe Precious Jeremiah

Abstract Substance use including alcohol, tobacco, prescription drugs, inhalants, and many others in sub-Saharan Africa and around the world has deleterious consequences on the health, economy, and social aspects of society. There is no single approach to dealing with substance use as intervention depends on aetiology, personality traits of the users, and the different rehabilitation services available. Thus, several strategies and multi-disciplinary approaches should be used for effective intervention.

K. L. Maikano (✉)
Legato Center for Psychometric Assessment, Gaborone, Botswana

R. P. Mogomotsi
Department of Psychology, University of Botswana, Gaborone, Botswana

K. Diraditsile
Waseda University, Shinjuku, Tokyo, Japan
e-mail: kabodira@fuji.waseda.jp

R. P. Jeremiah
Department of Social Work, University of Botswana, Gaborone, Botswana
e-mail: sinkambar@ub.ac.bw

M. Mhaka-Mutepfa (ed.), *Substance Use and Misuse in sub-Saharan Africa*, https://doi.org/10.1007/978-3-030-85732-5_11

The primary focus of this chapter is to explore and review prevention and effective interventions for harm reduction in substance use. Interventions for addressing problems that could not be prevented are discussed. The following interventions are discussed: cognitive-based therapies, confrontational models of intervention, crisis intervention, and systemic family models of persuasive intervention.

Keywords Effective intervention • Cognitive based therapy • Crisis intervention • Family model intervention • Psycho-education programs • Confrontational model intervention • Personality traits

Preventative Strategies of Substance Use Among Adults

The use of harmful substances, legal and illegal, presents substantial health risks and therefore prevention remains a priority (Lewer et al., 2019). Prevention of substance use in young people has been covered in detail in the previous chapter (Chap. 10). The methods used to prevent substance use in youths are not very different from those used in adults. What differs is the techniques stakeholders use when dealing with adults as adulthood has the highest rates of associated medical conditions (e.g., cancer, sexually transmitted infections, heart disease) and mental health conditions (e.g., bipolar, anxiety, and antisocial personality disorders) (Schulte & Hser, 2014).

Prevention of substance use, like any other prevention modality, falls into four stages: primordial prevention (e.g., policies banning tobacco marketing and built environment), primary prevention (e.g., cessation programs and immunisations), secondary prevention (e.g., substance use disorder (SUD) screening), and tertiary prevention (e.g., rehabilitation) (Kisling et al., 2021). A combination of these stages aims to prevent the onset of diseases through risk reduction, and long-term psychological (e.g., paranoia and depression) and medical conditions (e.g., liver cirrhosis and cancer) including SUDs (U.S. Department of Health and Human Services, 2016, pp. 3–1; Kisling et al., 2021) that may manifest later. As such, prevention of substance use needs the attention of all stakeholders (e.g., psychologists, social workers, medical doctors, psychiatrists, etc.) because of its widespread nature and high impact on individuals, families, and communities.

There are techniques and policies that can be put in place to prevent substance use and misuse. Programmes that are effective in preventing substance use and misuse include cognitive restructuring (which helps individuals recognise, challenge, and modify thought patterns and beliefs that support substance use) and community mobilisation (a programme that brings together multiple sectors to address substance use by assembling necessary resources, disseminating information, generating support, and fostering cooperation). Strategies and programmes that have proven to be effective have been discussed in Chap. 10. In addition to strategies and programmes, policy enforcement, laws, and regulations (primordial prevention) are also vital for prevention of access to substances (Substance Abuse and Mental Health Services Administration (SAMHSA, 2019).

Primordial Prevention Approaches

The policies pertaining to alcohol have been discussed in detail in Chap. 4. Additionally, policies pertaining to tobacco have been discussed in Chap. 6. However, it should be noted that it is easier to regulate taxes and prices for licit substances (International Drug Policy Consortium [IDPC], 2021) because the government can intervene. The foregoing authors also posited that in sub-Saharan Africa, illicit drugs cross borders without much detection as these cannot be regulated; thus efforts made to eradicate illicit drugs become overwhelming. More needs to be done in this area.

In addition to the programmes and policies that can aid in prevention of substance use and misuse, there are also primary prevention approaches.

Primary Prevention Approaches

The prevention approaches may include, among others, information dissemination, fear arousal, and resistance skills training.

Information Dissemination: This is mostly the first approach used to prevent the use and misuse of substances (tobacco, alcohol, prescription drugs, and illicit drugs). It encompasses efforts to increase understanding and awareness of the adverse health, social, and legal concerns of using one or more of these substances. This prevention approach includes public information campaigns by means of electronic and/or print media. Information dissemination is premised on the perception that people have inadequate knowledge on the adverse outcomes of using these substances and that once they are knowledgeable, they will develop negative attitudes towards the substances and minimise or stop using them (Botvin & Griffin, 2016).

Fear Arousal: Fear appeals is about arousing negative emotional reactions in order to promote self-protective motivation and action and is seen as a behaviour change method (Kok et al., 2016; 2018). This approach is frequently used in conjunction with information dissemination and is anticipated to discourage substance misuse by showcasing the negative consequences and symptoms of substance misuse in an effort to evoke fear or terror. Examples may include graphic pictures of cancerous lungs and auto fatalities resulting from driving under the influence of substances (Botvin & Griffin, 2016). The assumption is that when people are emotionally confronted with the negative effects of their behaviour (substance use and misuse), they may change their behaviour by either quitting or reducing intake of the substances (Kok et al., 2018). However, Ruiter et al. (2014) established that using fear arousal could in fact be counterproductive. They suggested that fear appeals may not be effective in behaviour change because people can just ignore the messages, minimise the severity of the threat due to desensitisation, and/or even deny the personal relevance of the threat.

Case Study 11.1: Persuasiveness of Fear Appeals

A study conducted by Shehryar and Hunt (2005) in the United States on terror management perspective on the persuasiveness of fear appeals indicated that participants with high-commitment to drinking who saw a death related appeal were significantly more likely to reject the intended message as compared to participants who saw the arrest and serious injury appeals. Overall, the fear tactic of showing participants the arrest and injury appeals proved to work as a preventative approach of substance misuse.

Stop and Reflect

1. Discuss why seeing is believing with regards to substance use and misuse.
2. Discuss why people may not be scared of dying from substance use and misuse.
3. In what way(s) can the threat (death) of the fear appeal be minimised by users?

Resistance Skills Training: This approach imparts skills for resisting peer and media influences to either smoke, drink, or use drugs. It is based on the idea that social influence plays a role in substance use and misuse (Botvin & Griffin, 2016). According to Botvin and Grifin (2016), social backgrounds impact substance use in at least two ways. First, social background associated with childhood development (family, peer relationships) influences drug use vulnerability. Factors influencing substance use include use by parents and exposure through social media. Second, the social setting also influences the functional effects of substance use, thereby directly impacting the fulfilment of substance intake behaviours (Botvin & Griffin, 2016). The foregoing suggest that substance use becomes a requirement for affiliation with selective groups and becomes a time out from social rules (Bardo et al., 2013).

Psychosocial Intervention Strategies

Substance use affects different aspects of people's lives such as the psychological, social, and financial aspects. In addition to the preventative strategies, intervention strategies may also be used to aid individuals in better managing their substance intake and assist those who have substance dependence to return to optimum functioning. There are numerous intervention strategies that may be employed to achieve these goals including pharmacological and psychosocial strategies. This chapter will focus on psychosocial strategies as pharmacological strategies have been discussed in Chap. 10.

Psychosocial intervention strategies are those that involve a qualified professional working with an individual to identify and manage their substance use/misuse and its consequent problems (USDHHS, 2016). It is important that these strategies be delivered by a qualified professional as the process of dealing with the substance use/misuse is a sensitive one in which a wrong move from the service provider could have detrimental effects on the individual. These could include the substance user withdrawing from the process, or even worsening the user's situation.

This intervention strategy may be delivered in several ways that differ according to the theoretical foundations they are built upon. These include the Cognitive Behavioural Therapies (CBTs), Motivational Interviewing (MI), Crisis Intervention (CI) Models, and Family Models of Intervention. The strategies are discussed below. Other psychosocial interventions that are conducted by para-professionals, non-professionals or users in recovery are not mentioned but they are also effective (e.g., Alcoholic Anonymous groups).

Cognitive Behavioural Therapies: Cognitive Behavioural Therapy (CBT) is a group of psychotherapies based on the learning theory that assumes a bidirectional relationship between behaviour and cognitive processes (McHugh et al., 2010; McLeod, 2019). According to the aforementioned authors, the different modalities under the CBT umbrella share the notion that the main purpose of therapy is to identify and assist the client in managing maladaptive patterns of behaviour, barriers to change that the client may be facing, and focusing on skills training. CBT views substance use as a maladaptive behaviour that is reinforced by the effects of the substances (Cleary et al., 2008). As such, therapeutic techniques are put in place to counteract the reinforcement of use and increase likelihood of the client not using the substances.

CBT is a structured, collaborative, time-limited intervention, with the number of sessions usually ranging from 1 session to 12 sessions (Jhanjee, 2014). There is an emphasis on CBT's structured nature as it is a skill building exercise on its own, teaching organising skills to the clients. The treatment process is structured into three phases (McHugh et al., 2010; McLeod, 2019). Phase 1 of the processes involves the assessment of the client's current functioning; this is done via screening tools and other psychometric assessments, and the treatment goals are also established at this phase. Furthermore, the phase involves performing a functional analysis as well as creating a case conceptualisation. A functional analysis is a process of understanding what purpose the client's actions are serving (Jhanjee, 2014). Case conceptualisation assists in using the CBT models to better organise and understand the client's symptoms, their background information, their presenting problem, as well as the factors influencing and maintaining the use of the substance. This process is vital as it helps to better understand the uniqueness of each client case and aids in building the best treatment plan for each client (McHugh et al., 2010; McLeod, 2019).

Phase 2 of the treatment process involves working on achieving the set treatment goals through use of cognitive and behavioural techniques and skills training sessions (McHugh et al., 2010; McLeod, 2019). Some of the techniques that may be used include cognitive reconstruction, thought challenging, and behavioural activation. In the final phase, outcome assessments are done, and focus is on consolidating the changes the client has undergone and skills they have learnt as well as working on relapse prevention. All sessions of CBT generally follow a similar session structure of reviewing the previous session, review of the homework given in previous session, outlining the current session's work, doing the session work, assigning homework, and review of the session (McHugh et al., 2010; McLeod, 2019). CBT is considered one of the most effective intervention strategies, even when dealing with comorbid psychological disorders (Parks et al., 2004). It is vital for readers to take cognisance of the fact that in CBT, cognitions (thoughts, beliefs, and/or interpretations) are the driving force behind behaviour. It is also important to note that intervention strategies like CBT can be done in groups.

Case Study 11.2: CBT for a Client with Alcohol Use Disorder

John is 27 years old and has struggled with alcohol use since he was 20. He was dismissed from his previous job as he would occasionally go to work intoxicated and on other days miss work. John reported that since the dismissal, he has withdrawn from his family and friends and resorted to daily drinking leaving him feeling worthless, guilty, and suicidal. Goals for psychotherapy were established, John's history was acquired, and assessments were done. Thought challenging and thought reconstructions were used to assist John to counter the feelings of guilt, worthlessness, and suicidal ideation. John was encouraged to think of alternative coping mechanisms. Situations were identified where he felt that he would be triggered to engage in alcohol use, the consequences of such relapses were discussed, and strategies were discussed of how best he could avoid relapse.

(K. Maikano, personal communication, October 20, 2020)

Stop and Reflect

1. What assessment could have been used to evaluate John's alcohol use?
2. Outline the process that was used for treatment.
3. Discuss any steps that were left out of the case study if any.

Motivational Interviewing: Motivational Interviewing (MI) is a collaborative counselling style that fosters behavioural change by assisting a client in working through the ambivalence they may be facing (Hettema et al., 2005) about their substance use/misuse. MI is a client-centred approach that balances the use of an empathic and supportive approach as well as a directive and confrontational approach to materialise the goals of treatment (Hettema et al., 2005). In MI, confrontation is used to facilitate change by focusing on the discrepancy between the client's values and goals and their current situation (Rollnick & Allison, 2004). There are four core principles of MI, for example, expressing empathy, supporting self-efficacy, progressing with resilience, and developing discrepancy, which guide the process of change during the delivery of the programme. Several models are used in implementing psychosocial intervention strategies.

Stages of Change Model: MI assumes that a client transitions through different stages of change as they go through the process of treatment. These five stages, as conceptualised (Prochaska & DiClemente, 2002; Prochaska & Norcross, 2002), are experienced by people as they make changes in their lives (Rollnick & Allison, 2004):

1. Precontemplation: Individuals in this stage may still be unaware of the negative consequences of their actions and as such do not intend on changing such behaviour at the time or in the foreseeable future.
2. Contemplation: Individuals are marked by the recognition of the negative consequences of their behaviour as they start to consider changing these behaviours, though they may still be unsure.
3. Preparation: At this stage, the individuals believe that change is the best option for them and they start planning towards that change.
4. Action: The individuals believe that they have the power to change their behaviours in this stage and begin to act towards changing their behaviour.
5. Maintenance: The individuals work towards maintaining the change they have made and avoiding relapse.

Despite research suggesting the efficacy of this approach in systematic analysis where 64% of the studies showed a moderate effect (Rubak, 2005) and a small effect (Zomahoun et al., 2016), MI is still an underutilised technique in sub-Saharan Africa. The underutilisation may be a consequence of contradicting findings where small significant valuable effects of MI were established in 7% (11 out of 155) of meta-analysis evaluations (Frost et al., 2018). However, underutilisation could also be due to lack of research concerning use of this method for treatment of substance use/misuse in low- and middle-income countries (LMICs). Thus, there is a need for more research on the strategy and more counsellors need to be trained in MI as unskilled use of MI could lead to unsuccessful treatment (Rollnick & Allison, 2004).

Crisis Intervention Models: Crisis Intervention (CI) is another strategy that may be used to assist clients with challenges relating to substance use/misuse. Crises may occur to anyone and at any time, disrupting the functionality or stability of the individual's life at that time. Thus, the aim of CI models is to provide an "emotional first aid" for the client and to help them build coping skills they can use in future (Dass-Brailsford, 2007). CI models comprise solution focused strategies that are brief as they focus on dealing with the client's current crisis; specific goals that can be attained in a short period are set at the beginning of the intervention. There are different models of CI that have unique defining features though they share the above-mentioned principles. Three of these models are discussed below:

Gilliland's Six Step Model: This model includes two steps, each with three aspects (Dass-Brailsford, 2007). These steps include the listening steps and the action steps. Listening steps include defining the situation, ensuring that the client is safe and providing support and the action steps include exploring alternatives, making plans, and attaining commitment (Dass-Brailsford, 2007).

Triage Assessment System: This is a model that assesses the crisis reaction of the client in three different domains, the cognitive, affective, and behavioural domains (Dass-Brailsford, 2007). The cognitive domain assesses the client's thinking while the affective domain assesses the client's emotions, and the behavioural domain assesses the client's actions. This model also focuses on the different areas of the client's life that may be affected by the crisis, and these include the individual's physical, social, psychological, and/or moral aspects of their lives (Dass-Brailsford, 2007).

Seven Stage Model: The seven steps of this model include (1) performing an extensive assessment that investigates the crisis, biopsychosocial aspects, suicidality, and homicidality risk, (2) building rapport with the client, (3) understanding the dimensions of the crisis, precipitating factors, and previous challenges, (4) eliciting and exploring client's feelings and emotions, (5) exploring how the client has coped with previous challenges, (6) establishing and implementing an action plan, and (7) planning for a follow-up session (Dass-Brailsford, 2007).

Case Study 11.3: Client with Alcohol Use Disorder
Jane is a 35-year-old mother of three. She has been periodically using alcohol and cannabis since her late teens. Jane reports that she has had challenges with depressive thoughts; alcohol and cannabis help her feel better, but the alcohol use has adversely affected her. Medical records have shown that Jane's physical health has been rapidly deteriorating and this is mainly linked to her substance use. With regards to her psychological functioning, Jane's feelings of guilt and inadequacy have weakened her mental well-being. Her interpersonal relationships have also been affected as her romantic relationship is currently strained.

(K. Maikano, personal communication, January 21, 2021).

Stop and Reflect

1. Discuss the similarities and differences in treatment in the three CI models.
2. Which would you prefer to use and why?

Systemic Family Models of Intervention: These models focus on how the family may be of assistance to the individual experiencing substance use/misuse challenges as well as how the family may influence the person's use or misuse of the substance. They view the individual as part of a family and as such, intervention does not only focus on the individual but the system as a whole (Rowe, 2012). Therapy sessions under these models aim to assess and tackle family issues that may have led the individual to use/

misuse substances and to help each member understand the role they play in the substance use/misuse and the strategies they may use to change these and prevent further issues (Rowe, 2012). The psychosocial interventions explored in this section aim to assist the individual to manage their substance use/misuse and achieving optimum functioning (Jhanjee, 2014). Besides having a common goal, these strategies also most commonly follow a similar protocol for the process. The universal protocol for the process of treatment involves assessing the individual's state and how the substance is affecting their life before creating a plan for treatment (USDHHS, 2016). This is referred to as the screening process, which is a secondary prevention approach.

Secondary Prevention Approaches

There are a number of screening tools that may be used during the screening process.

Screening for Substance Use/Misuse, Dependency, and Substance Use Disorders: This is generally the first step of the treatment process. It assists in identifying the individual's current state of functioning regarding the substance. This is important as it helps the mental health professional to tailor a treatment plan that may work best for the client (Henry-Edwards et al., 2003). Screening may also help the client to become more aware of how much the substance is affecting their life. A few screening tools that may be used include the following (see McPherson & Hersch, 2000):

Alcohol Use Disorders Identification Test (AUDIT): This 10-item screening tool was developed to identify individuals whose alcohol use may be putting them at danger (World Health Organisation, 2001). The AUDIT's primary aim is to identify frequency of use, dependency and the consequences of the alcohol consumption on the individual's life (Babor et al., 2001). The foregoing authors posit that the AUDIT may not be used to diagnose SUDs as per the diagnostic criteria. This tool may be administered by a professional or paraprofessional as a short oral interview or the individual may be asked to respond to the items in writing.

Addiction Severity Index (ASI): The ASI is a set of clinical interview questions that focus on seven aspects of the inividual's life and is designed to be administred orally by a professional. The ASI is most commonly used as an outcome measure to assess the impact of treatment for an individual.

Drug Abuse Screening Test (DAST): The DAST is a 28-item questionnaire used to screen for drug abuse as well as assess treatment outcome (Skinner, 1982). The tool has two other versions available for use (e.g., the 10-item shortened version and the 20-item version). As its main purpose is to screen for substance use, severity, and the consequences of use, it is usually paired with another screening tool that focuses more on alcohol use like the AUDIT (Skinner, 1982).

Alcohol, Smoking, and Substance Involvement Screening Test (ASSIST): The ASSIST is an eight-item questionnaire designed to be answered by the individual in writing to screen for a history of use in an individual's lifetime and within the preceding three months (see Newcombe et al., 2005). The test covers numerous substances and assesses harm, dependency, and the consequences of use for the individual. Other screening tools that are commonly used include the Substance Use Subtle Screening Inventory-Third Edition (SASSI-3), Severity of Dependence Scale (SDS), Maudsley Addiction Profile (MAP), and the Drug Use Screening Inventory (DUSI).

Tertiary Prevention Approaches

These strategies are applied in substance users who have SUDs or symptoms emanating from use or misuse and therefore aim to alleviate severity and any symptoms that may manifest later. Rehabilitation efforts are the most common and effective forms of tertiary prevention (Kisling et al., 2021).

Conclusion

The cost, time, and resource constraints on stakeholders may lead to overlooking of many preventive services for substance users. There is no one-size-fits all when dealing with substance use/misuse prevention and intervention among adults. Providing information to educate individuals about the dangerous effects of substance use/misuse may prevent SUDs and the same could be argued about the arousal of fear and resistance skills training. Similarly, the psychosocial intervention strategies discussed in this chapter could be effective in assisting adults struggling with SUDs. There is therefore need to carefully evaluate each prevention strategy in view of the individual, cultural, and other environmental contexts. Interventions should also aim at advocacy, psycho-education programmes, and increasing cognitive behavioural skills. Stakeholders need to keep track of all the latest information (including education, risks, and benefits) on prevention procedures and ensure all substance users and the public have access to appropriate and effective services.

End of Chapter Questions

1. Summarise the distinguishing features for each of the strategies discussed.
2. Which factors influence the choice of intervention?
3. Is there a need to make adaptations to the discussed interventions so that they are suited to the sub-Saharan African context? Explain your answer.
4. How would you address the problem of substance use disorders in your community?
5. In your own view, do you think substance use/misuse prevention is effective? Explain your answer.

Discussion Question

1. What key competencies should counsellors or qualified service providers have before attempting to implement any of the intervention styles?

References

Bardo, M. T., Neisewander, J. L., & Kelly, T. H. (2013). Individual differences and social influences on the neurobehavioral pharmacology of abused drugs. *Pharmacology Reviews, 65*, 255–290. https://doi.org/10.1124/pr.111.005124

Babor, T. F., Higgins-Biddle, J. C., Saunders, J. B., & Monteiro, M. G. (2001). *The alcohol use disorders identification test. Guideline for use in primary care.* World Health Organisation. https://www.dualdiagnosis.co.uk/uploads/documents/originals/AUDIT.pdf

Botvin, G. J., & Griffin, K. W. (2016). Prevention of substance abuse. In J. C. Norcross, G. R. VandenBos, D. K. Freedheim, & R. Krishnamurthy (Eds.), *APA handbook of clinical psychology: Applications and methods* (Vol. 3, pp. 485–509). American Psychological Association. https://doi.org/10.1037/14861-026

Cleary, M., Hunt, G. E., Matheson, S. L., Siegfried, N., & Walter, G. (2008). Psychosocial interventions for people with severe mental illnesses and substance misuse. *Cochrane Database of Systematic Reviews.* Jan 23;(1):CD001088. https://doi.org/10.1002/14651858.CD001088.pub2

Dass-Brailsford, P. (2007). *A practical approach to trauma: Empowering interventions.* Sage Publications.

Frost, H., Campbell, P., Maxwell, M., O'Carroll, R. E., Dombrowski, S. U., Williams, B., Cheyne, H., Coles, E., & Pollock, A. (2018). Effectiveness of motivational interviewing on adult behaviour change in health and social care settings: A systematic review of reviews. *PLoS One, 13*(10), e0204890. https://doi.org/10.1371/journal.pone.0204890.

Henry-Edwards, S., Humeniuk, R., Ali, R., Monteiro, M., & Poznyak, V. (2003). *Brief intervention for substance use: A manual for use in primary care* (Draft version 1.1 for field testing). World Health Organization.

Hettema, J., Steele, J., & Miller, W. R. (2005). Motivational interviewing. *The Annual Review of Clinical Psychology, 1*, 91–111. https://doi.org/annurev.clinpsy.1.102803.143833

International Drug Policy Consortium. (2021). *Policy and advocacy: Sub-Saharan Africa*. https://idpc.net/policy-advocacy/regional-work/sub-saharan-africa

Jhanjee, S. (2014). Evidence based psychosocial interventions in substance use. *Indian Journal of Psychological Medicine, 36*(2), 112–118.

Kisling, L. A., & Das, J. M. (2021). *Prevention strategies*. StatPearls Publishing. https://www.ncbi.nlm.nih.gov/books/NBK537222/

Kok, G., Gottlieb, N. H., Peters, G. J., Mullen, P. D., Parcel, G. S., Ruiter, R. A., & Bartholomew, L. K. (2016). A taxonomy of behavior change methods: An intervention mapping approach. *Health Psychology Review, 10*(3), 297–312. https://doi.org/10.1080/17437199.2015.1077155.

Kok, G., Peters, G. J. Y., Kessels, L. T., Hoor, G. A., & Ruiter, R. A. (2018). Ignoring theory and misinterpreting evidence: The false belief in fear appeals. *Health Psychology Review, 12*(2), 111–125. https://doi.org/10.1080/17437199.2017.1415767.

Lewer, D., Tweed, E. J., Alridge, R. W., & Morley, K. I. (2019). Causes of hospital admission and mortality among 6683 people who use heroin: A cohort study comparing relative and absolute risks. *Drug and Alcohol Dependence, 204*. https://doi.org/10.1016/j.drugalcdep.2019.06.027.

McHugh, K. R., Hearon, B. A., & Otto, M. W. (2010). Cognitive behavioral therapy for substance use disorders. *Psychiatric Clinics of North America, 33*(3), 511–525. https://doi.org/10.1016/j.psc.2010.04.012.

McLeod, S. (2019, January 11). *Cognitive behaviour therapy*. https://www.simplypsychology.org/cognitive-therapy.html

McPherson, T. L., & Hersch, R. K. (2000). Brief substance use screening instruments for primary care settings. *Journal of Substance Abuse Treatment, 18*(2), 193–202.

Newcombe, D. A., Humeniuk, R. E., & Ali, R. (2005). Validation of the World Health Organization alcohol, smoking and substance involvement screening test (ASSIST): Report of results from the Australian site. *Drug and Alcohol Review, 24*(3), 217–226.

Parks, G. A., Marlatt, G. A., & Anderson, B. K. (2004). Cognitive-behavioral alcohol treatment. In N. Heather & T. Stockwell (Eds.), *The essential handbook of treatment and prevention of alcohol problems* (pp. 69–86). John Wiley & Sons Ltd.

Prochaska, J. O., & DiClemente, C. C. (2002). Transtheoretical therapy. In F. W. Kaslow & J. Lebow (Eds.), *Comprehensive handbook of psychotherapy* (Integrative/Eclectic) (Vol. 4, pp. 165–183). Wiley.

Prochaska, J. O., & Norcross, J. C. (2002). Stages of change. In J. C. Norcross (Ed.), *Psychotherapy relationships at work* (pp. 303–313). Oxford University Press.

Rollnick, S., & Allison, J. (2004). Motivational interviewing. In N. Heather & T. Stockwell (Eds.), *The essential handbook of treatment and prevention of alcohol problems* (pp. 105–115). John Wiley & Sons, Ltd.

Rubak, S., Sandbæk, A., Lauritzen, T., & Christensen, B. (2005). Motivational interviewing: a systematic review and meta-analysis. *British journal of general practice, 55*(513), 305–312.

Rowe, C. L. (2012). Family therapy for drug abuse: Review and updates 2003–2010. *Journal of Marital & Family Therapy, 38*(1), 59–81. https://doi.org/10.1111/j.1752-0606.2011.00280.x.

Ruiter, R. A., Kessels, L. T., Peters, G. J. Y., & Kok, G. (2014). Sixty years of fear appeal research: Current state of the evidence. *International Journal of Psychology, 49*, 63–70. https://doi.org/10.1002/ijop.12042.

SAMHSA. (2019). *Substance misuse prevention for young adults.* Substance Abuse and Mental Health Services Administration.

Schulte, M. T., & Hser, Y. (2014). Substance use and associated health conditions throughout the lifespan. *Public Health Reviews, 35*(2), 1–27.

Shehryar, O., & Hunt, D. M. (2005). A terror management perspective on the persuasiveness of fear appeals. *Journal of Consumer Psychology, 15*(4), 275–287.

Skinner, H. A. (1982). The drug abuse screening test. *Addictive Behaviors, 7*(4), 363–371. https://doi.org/10.1016/0306-4603(82)90005-3.

U.S. Department of Health and Human Services. (2016). *Facing addiction in America: The surgeon general's report on alcohol, drugs, and health.* Substance Abuse and Mental Health Services Administration.

World Health Organisation. (2001). *AUDIT The Alcohol Use Disorders Identification Test: Guidelines for use in primary health care.* World Health Organisation. https://www.who.int/publications-detail-redirect/audit-the-alcohol-use-disorders-identification-test-guidelines-for-use-in-primary-health-care

Zomahoun, H. T. V., Guénette, L., Grégoire, J.-P., Lauzier, S., Lawani, A. M., Ferdynus, C., & Moisan, J. (2016). Effectiveness of motivational interviewing interventions on medication adherence in adults with chronic diseases: A systematic review and meta-analysis. *International Journal of Epidemiology, 46*(2), 589–602. https://doi.org/10.1093/ije/dyw273.

CHAPTER 12

Conclusion

Magen Mhaka-Mutepfa and James January

Abstract Substance use disorders contribute immensely to the global burden of disease. In this final chapter, overviews of the book chapters are summarized and the key points have been highlighted. In the first section of the book, major factors that contribute to the causation, risks, signs, and symptoms of substance use/misuse as well as mental and behavioural disorders emanating from the commonly used substances in the sub-Saharan African region were discussed. In the second section, an exposition of prevention, treatment, and intervention of substance use and misuse within the sub-Saharan Africa context was presented. The chapter also highlights the interventions and possible challenges that may arise when instituting interventions to curb substance use disorders. The last section of this chapter addresses implications for research, practice, and policy in light of substance use disorders in Africa.

M. Mhaka-Mutepfa (✉)
Department of Psychology, Faculty of Social Sciences, University of Botswana, Gaborone, Botswana
e-mail: mutepfam@ub.ac.bw

J. January
Department of Community Medicine, College of Health Sciences, University of Zimbabwe, Harare, Zimbabwe
e-mail: jamesj@medsch.uz.ac.zw

M. Mhaka-Mutepfa (ed.), *Substance Use and Misuse in sub-Saharan Africa*, https://doi.org/10.1007/978-3-030-85732-5_12

Keywords Substance use disorders • Causation • Mental and behavioural disorders • Challenges • Implications

Substance use related problems continue to pose serious public health challenges the world over. Thus, it is imperative that appropriate evidence-based interventions be developed and instituted to curb the growing burden of substance use and misuse especially in resource-limited settings such as much of sub-Saharan Africa. The previous chapters in this book provide a summary of pertinent issues in understanding the substance use/misuse in the sub-Saharan African region.

The first section of this book gives an exposition of the causes, risk factors, signs, and symptoms of substance use/misuse as well as mental and behavioural disorders emanating from the commonly used substances in the region. The signs and symptoms of substance use disorders (SUDs) vary among individuals depending on the type of substance ingested and the individual's personal and social situations. For instance, personal circumstances such as loneliness can lead to diverse mental, physical, and social effects to people with SUDs which may affect them and their significant others' quality of life and wellbeing (Mhaka-Mutepfa et al., 2021). On the other hand, stressful and adverse events that can lead to substance use/misuse can exacerbate already existing psychological problems (e.g., depression and anxiety), thus the need for early effective intervention.

The adverse effects of substances on individuals have been demonstrated clearly in literature by numerous researchers (e.g., Diraditsile & Rasesigo, 2018; Kisling et al., 2021). Thus, over the years we have come to know that the use and misuse of substances result in a plethora of other health problems. However, despite the knowledge of these harmful consequences, the habit of ingesting substances still continues. Despite the existence of evidence suggesting that the use of illegal substances can lead to bodily damage and complications with blood vessels (Felman, 2018), people are still not perturbed. In addition, the abrupt stoppage of a substance can result in physiological symptoms (e.g., withdrawal), and/or social effects (e.g., giving up social engagements). In some cases, individuals may continue taking the substance despite the adverse effects. For instance, a person with alcohol use disorder may continue drinking even after being diagnosed with liver cirrhosis and continue to take the substance in order to feel good and dull the pain. Legal difficulties may also ensue since substances can impair judgement or increase risks for behaviours such as public violence, or breaking the law to access the substance. For expensive substances, financial difficulties may arise.

There is a particular need to pay greater attention to younger populations in the fight against substance use and misuse. Previous research has documented evidence supporting the notion that when consumption of substances begins at an early age, the ramifications are more serious (Stormshak et al., 2014). For instance, youth aged 15 years and below who initiate consistent substance use are at increased risk of dependency and associated diseases of lifestyle such as sexually transmitted infections, HIV and AIDS, liver disorders, type 2 diabetes, and cardiovascular conditions. Apart from increasing morbidity and mortality, use of substances is also associated with decreased and impaired brain functioning which negatively impacts learning, motivation, and memory as the drugs cause neurotransmitter imbalances, particularly dopamine and serotonin (Toumbourou et al., 2007).

While exposure to substances at a young age has been shown to contribute immensely to drug dependency, there are other factors which also increase the deleterious effects of substances. Stressful early life experiences such as being abused or suffering other forms of trauma are some of the important risk factors in the aetiology of substance use disorders and those with a history of physical and/or sexual abuse are more likely to be diagnosed with SUDs (Tonmyr & Shields, 2017). Other pertinent risk factors include genetic vulnerability, prenatal exposure to alcohol or other drugs, lack of parental supervision or monitoring, social learning and modelling from family members who are users and association with drug-using peers also play an important role.

Interventions for Addressing Substance Use and Misuse

The second section of this book gives an exposition of prevention, treatment and intervention of substance use and misuse within the sub-Saharan Africa context. Due to the significant costs associated with substance use/misuse, prevention efforts (primordial, primary, secondary, and tertiary) should be paramount in addressing this growing burden. However, there have been concerns from other stakeholders on whether these prevention efforts are indeed worthwhile. Sinkamba (2015), for example, argued that regardless of the existing intervention strategies, the use of substances such as alcohol continues to escalate. One plausible explanation for this could be that there appears to be a lack of comprehensive and coordinated attempts to engage in critical analyses on why there is a rising trend in substance usage despite various mitigation efforts (e.g., policy interventions by governments). There is need to, therefore, tackle this problem using multi-sectoral and multi-disciplinary approaches.

Parental and family programmes aimed at assisting families raise children in more secure and responsible environments (Kumpfer & Alvarado, 2003) have shown some efficacy in reducing the problem of substance use is some settings. Where such programs are effected, continuous monitoring and evaluating is needed. Interventions also need to be tailor-made for the targeted groups since there is no "one size fits all" approach. Thus, opportunities should be availed in sub-Saharan African settings to further develop novel interventions and continue to test existing ones.

Interventions for substance use and misuse have mostly taken the form of behavioural therapy. There is, however, a need to consider a broader spectrum of antecedents that may be contributing to the problem through the use of a biopsychosocial approach. Such an approach would ensure that the individual's developmental stage, cognitive abilities, family, and societal contexts are taken into consideration when addressing the presenting problem.

Challenges of the Interventions

It is clear from the foregoing discussion that although most interventions have made some modest achievements towards tackling substance use/misuse, evidence shows that the challenges far outweigh the successes. Available programme data based on evidence from the field, anecdotes and observations suggest that, over the years, substance use/misuse interventions, inclusive of policies, have experienced a few challenges and as such have not fully succeeded in achieving their core mandate. For example, some of the alcohol policies in different countries do not pronounce the composition of the inter-sectoral committees in terms of the required level of authority of its members (e.g., the Botswana alcohol policy). Tapera et al. (2020) posited that in Botswana, for instance, with only six officers at national level and no structures or representatives at district level, the committee is too small, given the magnitude of the alcohol problem and the complexity of socio-economic, cultural, and other factors underlying it. There is, therefore, a need for governments to empower and strengthen these inter-sectoral committees by formalizing their terms of reference (TORs), although it should be noted that the TORs alone may not be sufficient to empower the committees to provide effective "strategic guidance, coordination and supervision of the national policies" (United Nations Development Program, 2017).

These challenges should be looked into to curb SUD problems and implications for research, practice and policy should also be discussed.

Implications for Research, Practice, and Policy

Substance use/misuse and its abundant problems is a continuous challenge for stakeholders (e.g., governments and civic society, social workers, health personnel, etc.). The literature presented in this book serves as an evidence base that can be used to inform stakeholders, inclusive of policy makers about interventions that have been piloted as well as highlighting significant areas for future research. For the widespread substance use/misuse challenges to be addressed, more emphasis should be on further research to generate on-going, valid, and reliable evidence that may provide answers to the omnipresent problem of substance use/misuse.

The authors concur that more research is needed, particularly focusing more on the effectiveness of prevention and intervention strategies used in mitigating substance use/misuse in order to establish evidence about efficacy. Thus, more research needs to be conducted to accurately estimate the extent of substance use disorders, and the efficacy of the intervention strategies that are in place. Although stakeholders may plan holistic and specialist approaches for practice and policy, implementation may be problematic. However, the shift from face-to-face treatment to telehealth has increased the use of SUD services (Abramson, 2021) and these can be continued for those with internet and telephone services even after COVID-19.

At practice level, needs assessment could provide useful baseline information for formulating efficacious interventions suitable for sub-Saharan countries. Interventions could be tailor-made for specific settings (e.g., interventions in prison, place of work, health-care settings as well as school- and family-based programmes) (Pistone et al., 2020). During practice, interventions also differ, for instance, there are technology-based interventions (e.g., mobile applications, web-based programmes, and text messages), and physical activities (e.g., workouts for children, yoga, and mindfulness for adults); thus, professionals should establish and apply interventions most suitable for the arena, individual, group or incidence. A combination of interventions (for instance, combining laws, enforcements, and restrictions or combining media campaigns, community education, telephone interviews, advertisements, and equality perspectives) can be used.

Family-based prevention programmes that focus on education, skills training, and resilience improvement to increase positive outcomes through reduction of risk factors should be introduced and strengthened (Kumpfer & Hansen, 2014). The family-based prevention programmes impart parenting and interpersonal skills and thus strengthen behaviours that intensify attachment, effective monitoring and communication, and disciplinary skills. There is ample evidence to suggest that the abovementioned protective factors are profound in shaping adolescents' substance taking behaviour as they directly impact on behaviours such as delinquency as well as academic achievement and other aspects such as teen pregnancy (Kumpfer & Alvarado, 2003). Support for family-based skills training programmes and their positive outcomes when addressing substance use/misuse among the youth abound (Foxcroft & Tsertsvadze, 2012; Kumpfer & Hansen, 2014) as they allow family members to learn and practice new skills together, which in turn enhances their communication and interactions.

At policy level, political and policy emphasis on all aspects of substance use/misuse should be intensified; it is paramount that professionals remain up-to-date on current issues and their responsibilities. Although some countries have implemented certain policies on substance use/misuse (e.g., alcohol and tobacco tax policies), they have failed to embrace WHO's tobacco control policies (i.e., the four regulatory categories; price, taxation, availability, marketing, and drink-driving measures) that are cost-effective (Morojele et al., 2021). More needs to be done in this area, especially engaging governments through robust advocacy to increase awareness of the long-term benefits of such policies. Additionally, interventions like MPOWER (Implemented by WHO to reduce smoking-attributable deaths by: **M**onitoring tobacco use prevention policies; **P**rotecting people from tobacco smoke; **O**ffering help for quitting tobacco use; **W**arning people about the dangers of tobacco; **E**nforcing bans on tobacco advertising, promotion and sponsorship; and **R**aising tobacco taxes.) (see Chap. 6) should be monitored and evaluated by establishing policy provisions in all countries. WHO can lead countries to make the policies effective and easy to implement.

Policies should also provide for the decentralization of the anti-alcohol, anti-tobacco, and anti-illicit substance responses to ensure there are district and community structures for dealing with substance use and misuse. Even though policies prioritize community action, the policies assume that communities will initiate actions on their own and collaborate with various agencies such as the police and other law-enforcement agencies to enforce response action without a focused, targeted coordinating structure. Governments should put up structures to initiate effective actions and these should be monitored and evaluated by multi-disciplinary teams for efficacy. Failure to do this will inevitably result in threats to public health and sustainable human development in Africa.

References

Abramson, A. (2021, March 1). *Substance use during the pandemic.* https://www.apa.org/monitor/2021/03/substance-use-pandemic

Diraditsile, K., & Rasesigo, K. (2018). Substance abuse and mental health effects among the youth in Botswana: Implications for social research. *Journal of Education, Society and Behavioural Science, 24*(2), 1–11.

Felman, A. (October 26, 2018). *What are the symptoms of addiction?* https://www.medicalnewstoday.com/articles/323459

Foxcroft, D. R., & Tsertsvadze, A. (2012). Universal alcohol misuse prevention programmes for children and adolescents: Cochrane systematic reviews. *Perspectives in Public Health, 132*, 128–134.

Kisling, L.A., & Das, J. M. (2021). *Prevention strategies.* StatPearls Publishing. Available from: https://www.ncbi.nlm.nih.gov/books/NBK537222/

Kumpfer, K. L., & Alvarado, R. (2003). Family-strengthening approaches for the prevention of youth problem behaviors. *American Psychologist, 58*(6-7), 457–465. https://doi.org/10.1037/0003-066X.58.6-7.457

Kumpfer, K. L., & Hansen, W. (2014). Family-based prevention programs. In L. Scheier & W. Hansen (Eds.), *Parenting and teen drug use* (pp. 166–192). Oxford Press.

Mhaka-Mutepfa, M., Biswas, A. J., Mfolwe, L., Mathoote, K., & Hasan, M. T. (2021). Well-being, loneliness, and quality of relationships before and during the COVID-19 pandemic in Botswana: Findings from cross-sectional analysis. *Manuscript submitted for publication.*

Morojele, N. K., Dumbili, E. W., Obot, I. S., & Parry, C. (2021). Alcohol consumption, harms and policy developments in sub-Saharan Africa: The case for stronger national and regional responses. *Drug and Alcohol Review, 40*(3), 402–419.

Pistone, I., Blomberg, A., & Sager, M. (2020). A systematic mapping of substance use, misuse, abuse and addiction prevention research: Current status and implications for future research. *Journal of Substance Use, 25*(3), 231–237. https://doi.org/10.1080/14659891.2019.1684583

Sinkamba, R. (2015). Alcohol abuse and interventions strategies in Botswana and China: A preliminary study. *Journal of African Studies, 29*(1), 157–170.

Stormshak, E. A., Connell, A. M., & al, M.-H.V. (2014). An ecological approach to promoting early adolescent mental health and social adaptation: Family-centered intervention in public middle schools. *Child Development, 82*(1), 209–225.

Tapera, R., Mbongwe, B., Mhaka-Mutepfa, M., Lord, A., Phaladze, N. A., & Zetola, N. M. (2020). The theory of planned behavior as a behavior change model for tobacco control strategies among adolescents in Botswana. *PLoS One, 15*(6). https://doi.org/10.1371/journal.pone.0233462.

Tonmyr, L., & Shields, M. (2017). Childhood sexual abuse and substance abuse: A gender paradox? *Child Abuse & Neglect, 63*, 284–294. https://doi.org/10.1016/j.chiabu.2016.11.004.

Toumbourou, J., Stockwell, T., Neighbors, C., Marlatt, G., Sturge, J., & Rehm, J. (2007). Interventions to reduce harm associated with adolescent substance use. *The Lancet, 369*(9570), 1391–1401.

United Nations Development Program. (2017). *Desk review of the Botswana National Alcohol Policy*. United Nations Development Program. https://www.moh.gov.bw/news_events/alcohol_consultation.html

Index

M. Mhaka-Mutepfa (ed.), *Substance Use and Misuse in sub-Saharan Africa*, https://doi.org/10.1007/978-3-030-85732-5

The manufacturer's authorised representative in the EU is Springer Nature Customer Service Centre GmbH, Europaplatz 3, 69115 Heidelberg, Germany. If you have any concerns regarding our products, please contact ProductSafety@springernature.com

Printed and bound by CPI Group (UK) Ltd, Croydon, CR0 4YY

30/09/2026

02225704-0001